AUTONOMY AND LONG-TERM CARE

AUTONOMY AND LONG-TERM CARE

George J. Agich

New York   Oxford
OXFORD UNIVERSITY PRESS
1993

Oxford University Press

Oxford   New York   Toronto
Delhi   Bombay   Calcutta   Madras   Karachi
Kuala Lumpur   Singapore   Hong Kong   Tokyo
Nairobi   Dar es Salaam   Cape Town
Melbourne   Auckland   Madrid

and associated companies in
Berlin   Ibadan

Published by Oxford University Press, Inc.,
200 Madison Avenue, New York, New York 10016

Oxford is a registered trademark of Oxford University Press

Library of Congress Cataloging-in-Publication Data
Agich, George J., 1947–
Autonomy and long-term care / George J. Agich.
p. cm.   Includes bibliographical references and index.
ISBN 0-19-507495-5
1. Aged—Long-term care—Moral and ethical aspects.   2. Autonomy
(Psychology) in old age.   3. Autonomy (Philosophy)   I. Title.
[DNLM: 1. Ethics, Medical.   2. Long-Term Care—in old age.
3. Long-Term care—psychology.   4. Patient Participation.
5. Professional-Patient Relations.   WT 30 A26458a]
RC954.3.A44 1993   174'.2—dc20
DNLMDLC for Library of Congress
92-49361

1 3 5 7 9 8 6 4 2

Printed in the United States of America

on acid-free paper

For Jackie and Pete,
Who see it from the inside

Preface

I began thinking about the problem of autonomy in the context of long-term care in a serious way in 1987 as I worked to develop a phenomenological framework for the ethics of long-term care. This research forced me to confront some of the difficulties associated with the meaning and function of autonomy in long-term care and led me to argue for an alternative to the mainstream, liberal view of autonomy. Readers of this work pressed for broadening the focus from long-term care in order to develop the implications of my views for medical ethics in general. I resisted those suggestions partly because the thrust of the suggested reorientation entailed writing a rather different book and also because I could not envision expanding the work to draw the implications for medical ethics without engaging the even wider philosophical questions related to the justification of autonomy. Given the observations of these astute readers, it might be helpful to explain the work's lineage as a way to make clear the work's relatively restricted focus.

This book grew from work originally begun under a grant from the Retirement Research Foundation's Personal Autonomy and Longterm Care Initiative in 1987–88. The funded project was itself the surviving part of a larger, collaborative proposal to study the social reality of autonomy in long-term care. This latter project had three interrelated objectives: to develop a theoretical framework for examining actions and behaviors of individuals and institutional practices that enhance or thwart autonomy of elders in long-term care, to develop an intervention designed to increase awareness in staff and elders of the complex dimensions of human existence that bear on respect for persons in long-term care settings, and to conduct qualitative and quantitative empirical research to evaluate the attitudes, behaviors, or beliefs in long-term care settings that might enhance or efface autonomy and to determine which might be amenable to modification.

The present work was thus originally conceived to have practical clinical implications. Although the framework developed is mainly conceptual, it is intended to support practical and empirical conclusions and further research. Understanding this objective is important since the argument advanced is that autonomy should be understood phenomenologically; the focus should be on concrete or actual (rather than abstract) autonomy. I argue that autonomy should be understood dispositionally, that is, in a comprehensive sense that defines the overall course of a person's life, rather than occurrently, the sense that is intended when we simply speak of people acting autonomously in a particular circumstance or situation. Only this dispositional or comprehensive sense of autonomy allows an individual to enjoy a life that is unified, orderly, and free from self-defeating conflict over fundamental values and beliefs.

I have borrowed rather freely, though selectively, from the gerontological literature. I can hardly claim expertise in this field, though my perusal of the literature has confirmed, at least to my own satisfaction, that my approach finds support—and in some instances finds inspiration—in the qualitative sociological literature on nursing home life and human life-span development.

My goal was to assess the prospects of and place for the concept of autonomy in an ethics of long-term care, not to catalog or treat exhaustively the problems of autonomy in long-term care. Other authors have taken this latter tack, but none, to my knowledge, have tried to forge a theory of autonomy in long-term care. I argue that autonomy is a central ethical concept for long-term care, but only if the understanding of autonomy is radically modified. I came to this conclusion after being struck by the ethical salience of a wide range of gerontological research, for example, on communication style and language, and the relative paucity and thinness of the self-proclaimed ethical work in this field. This impression sustained my effort to find a way to accommodate theoretically the qualitative gerontological research and to extend its insights for ethics of long-term care. Although I believe this work has implications—important ones, I hope—for the taxonomy of ethical problems and issues in long-term care on the one hand and for the practical ethics of long-term care on the other, the reader will have to look elsewhere for these implications to be drawn out. The limited focus of the present work permitted only suggestion of some general lines of application. Although the account I develop is practical, it nonetheless is primarily programmatic in intent and scope. The analysis and discussion will at certain points appear rather coarse-grained, leaving out much relevant detail. There are two reasons for this programmatic character.

First, the empirical and existential intricacy of long-term care precludes a comprehensive analysis given the limited scope of the present work. One should not expect detailed treatment of specific classes of long-term care; instead, the discussion proceeds by way of illustrative and paradigmatic examples. I reference the rich sociological and anthropological literature on aging and long-term care as it fills out the picture that is outlined here, though I am aware, perhaps more than my reader might ever be, of what more could have been said. Second, the ethical theory underlying the approach taken, a theory articulated, but only partly justified, consists in giving human judgment a central place. As a result, there is little in the way of prescriptions or rules to guide conduct; instead, a framework for rethinking and reconsidering the everyday ethics of long-term care is offered. For such a framework to have any practical significance requires that moral agents adopt its vantage point to inform their action. I could easily promise more, but fulfilling such a promise would be futile indeed.

The analysis of social action and the world of everyday life that occupies Chapter 5 is phenomenologically inspired. Sources for this analysis were diverse, ranging from philosophical phenomenological work to concrete existential and sociological studies. I have chosen to spare the reader much of the theoretical and methodological detail of phenomenological philosophy because it is widely available elsewhere and only ancillary to the main theme of this work. There seemed to be no manageable way to broach the subject with adequacy and retain the focus on the twin themes of autonomy and long-term care. I have acknowledged, as much as was practicable, my debt to philosophical phenomenology as well as to the anthropological and sociological ethnographic work that seems to carry out Alfred Schutz's program of a phenomenology of the social world (1967). If actual autonomy is a viable focus for ethics, then philosophers must give the phenomenology of the social world of everyday life far greater attention than has heretofore occurred.

Several points form the point of departure and rationale for this work. First, the literature on autonomy (and related discussions of paternalism and beneficence) seems to rely on a model of the patient regarded as a competent individual capable of acting and deciding in a rational and free fashion in terms of his or her own best interest. To be sure, concern has been expressed regarding these assumptions, but the assumptions are widely made and uncritically accepted by most authors. As mentioned above, my argument is not unrelated to these concerns, but the relationship can only be said to be tangential.

Second, I found very little literature helpfully dealing with the practical problems of respecting or enhancing the autonomy of the elderly in long-term care with one exception. That exception consists in the literature that focuses on the decisions to institutionalize, to initiate aggressive treatments, or to withhold and withdraw life-sustaining treatments focusing on the various rights of institutionalized elders. These treatments naturally flow from the standard understanding of autonomy in medical ethics. For my purposes, however, these treatments run in the wrong direction; they attend to specific decisions and choices that, though important, are only nodes in the dynamic and complex reality of long-term care.

Third, my review of the gerontological literature did not reveal any wide appreciation of the problems associated with autonomy; autonomy simply does not figure as a central research theme. There is, however, a good deal of practical attention to a variety of problems of long-term care that are relevant to the standard understanding of autonomy, even though this literature does not regularly utilize the language of ethics or autonomy—for example, work on communication styles between caregivers and elders, the phenomena of agitation, confusion, loneliness, or wandering among institutionalized elders, as well as the problems of providing emotional support and developing intervention techniques for impaired elders.

Fourth, I believe that an adequate understanding of the nature of human autonomy requires the incorporation of a developmental perspective, a perspective that is generally absent in most treatments. This absence partly helps explain why the problem of autonomy in the care of elders is primarily conceived as a problem of decisionmaking because elders are assumed to be fully formed selves with mature decision-making capacities. Hence, the emotional and psychosocial aspects of being old and impaired tend to be regarded as irrelevant or, at best, tangential to autonomy. A developmental orientation, however, provides strong evidence that this view is mistaken.

One difficulty associated with using the language of development in the context of long-term care was pointed out by an astute reviewer of an early draft. This reviewer complained that using a developmental perspective to defend what I call a parentalist position with respect to the care of frail or seriously incapacitated elders is perverse. Such talk struck this reviewer as importing misleading analogies (those from childhood) into long-term care and committing the gerontological sin of infantilizing elders. Spurred by these comments, I have tried to make my view of the significance of human development for the ethics of long-term care clearer than it apparently was in that early draft.

The task that I set for myself in this work, then, was to press the concept of autonomy into service as a fundamental ethical principle in understanding long-term care. To be sure, other ethical principles and considerations are relevant and important besides autonomy, though none enjoy a more central place in contemporary ethical thought.

If one is interested in developing a concept or a theory of autonomy, then one is primarily interested in "being autonomous," with the question "what does it mean to be autonomous?" However, if one is concerned with policies or practices designed to respect people's autonomy, then it is the "exercise of autonomy" that is central. Most philosophers seem concerned with the importance of being autonomous, not with practical ethical questions of promoting or enhancing the exercise of autonomy. This book, however, is concerned primarily with the latter question in the context of long-term care. Nevertheless, some discussion of the former question, namely, of theories and concepts of autonomy, was unavoidable. To some readers this may appear quaintly or objectionably "philosophical" and academic; these questions, however, cannot be bypassed and are considered just because these concepts infect the very practice of autonomy itself, particularly in the context of long-term care.

I venture a critical analysis and discussion of some of the complex philosophical treatments of autonomy only insofar as necessary to disentangle the practical and ethical questions of what it means to exercise autonomy. The risks in this strategy is that some readers will see the work as too philosophical, too theoretical, and will be dismayed by its failure to accommodate fully the vast empirical gerontological literature; others will see my treatment of vexatious conceptual and theoretical questions associated with autonomy as superficial.

To the first set of readers I can only say that my line of analysis and argument is exemplary of a method that itself deserves, perhaps requires, further methodological and theoretical treatment. Those readers might take solace in knowing that I have spared them that discussion. To those who might see the conceptual analysis and treatment of certain stock issues associated with autonomy as unsatisfying, I can say that this work represents something of a departure, though certainly not an entirely new one, from standard philosophical fare. The concept of actual exercise of autonomy that plays a central role in my treatment of long-term care has, I think, implications for a more traditional, theoretical philosophical work on what it means to be autonomous. My unwillingness to discuss fully contemporary philosophical treatments has already been explained above. I do think that the concept of actual autonomy might prove fruitful in its own right as a central concept of ethics; my treatment of it has been constrained, just as it was motivated, by my access through the practical problems associated with long-term care. I am indebted, probably more than my bibliography demonstrates, to recent work on autonomy and ethics which I regard as remarkably rich and valuable, especially given the rather thin amount of descriptive content that feeds that theoretical enterprise.

Some readers might wish for a more expanded treatment of relevant sociological and ethnographic gerontological literature. I would be the first to acknowledge that the phenomenological observations comprising Chapter 5, for example, could be further developed by fuller reference to qualitative gerontological studies. In this regard, I am guided more by the philosopher's than the gerontologist's interests and, perhaps, instincts. My intent is to develop a framework for *thinking* about what it means to exercise autonomy and what it means to respect autonomy in long-term care. I am concerned with constructing an orientation that will suggest new ways to conceptualize the practical ethical dimensions of long-term care or, perhaps, to place already-known truths and observations about long-term care in a different light.

Autonomy and the practical ethical problems that autonomy poses in long-term care thus provide my compass and map. My contribution is less that of an explorer charting new terrain or a cartographer surveying land with precision, than a teacher in the art of orienteering, of finding one's way through the terrain of long-term care guided by one's map and compass of autonomy.

I gratefully acknowledge the support of the Retirement Research Foundation for the initial work on this project as well as the opportunities to interact with other grantees under its Personal Autonomy and Longterm Care Initiative several times a year during the tenure of my award. Participants in the meetings of the grantees of the Personal Autonomy Initiative contributed greatly to expanding my appreciation of the practical difficulties of long-term care and helped to shape my own ideas. They will appreciate that I proved an attentive auditor of their presentations and discussions. I am also grateful for their critical comments and questions about my work. Discussions with Chuck Lidz over the years helped refine my own rather rough and ready intuitions about ethnographic research and some aspects of long-term care research as well. Reviewers of the prospectus and sample chapters I submitted to Oxford University Press provided trenchant critical comments that proved helpful on particular points, and confirmed the sensibility of the approach I had taken. In this regard, I would be remiss if I did not publicly acknowledge the incisive comments offered by Rick Moody on the original submission. I am much in his debt for calling to my attention several important questions and concerns that might otherwise have been glossed over. Transcription of the original report from which this book is drawn was ably accomplished by Melinda Weinrich; subsequent changes and drafts were typed by Beverly Bradley. Finally, my wife, Mary Kate Fredriksen, and son, Nicholas Agich, had to endure my absence or preoccupation during much of the holiday season of 1991 and January 1992 as the final revisions were completed. Their loving support and understanding is very deeply appreciated.

Springfield, Ill.   G.J.A.
June 1992

Contents

AUTONOMY AND LONG-TERM CARE

1

Introduction

The conjunction of autonomy and long-term care is remarkably paradoxical. Elders need long-term care because they suffer illnesses and incapacities that compromise their ability to function independently. Yet the standard concept of autonomy in bioethics stresses the values of independence and rational free-choice, values that seem rather ephemeral in the face of the wide range of impairments that cause elders to seek long-term care. No doubt such individuals are vulnerable and so might benefit from the protection afforded by autonomy-derived rights such as noninterference. The paradox nonetheless remains in that autonomy supports a concept of persons as robust and independent, whereas the reality of long-term care shows individuals who need support and companionship, needs that seem inimical to this ideal of autonomy. The paradox thus involves the contrast between the independence central to standard views of autonomy and the dependence that inescapably characterizes long-term care. Underlying this paradox is a standard view of autonomy that involves a rather abstract concept of human persons and agency.

Autonomy as traditionally conceived in the liberal tradition focuses on independence of action, speech, and thought. It provides the broad foundation for a wide range of political, legal, civil, and human rights that are designed to ensure that individuals are able to resist the coercive interference of any external authority or power in their own lives. The ideals implicit in this concept of autonomy include independence and self-determination, the ability to make rational and free decisions, and an ability to accurately assess what constitutes the individual's own best interest. This concept of autonomy has led to worries about paternalism, the use of (varying degrees of) coercion to impose another's vision—where the other might be the state, private institutions, or individuals—on a single individual or class of individuals. The concept of autonomy so understood supports a set of values such as independence and self-determination that have provided the normative standards around which tyranny, oppression, and even the benevolent use of power over vulnerable individuals have been opposed.

3

If we approach the task of enhancing the autonomy of elders in long-term care from a critical appreciation of this tradition, an occlusion becomes obvious that requires attention. Autonomy and long-term care are each rather diffuse cultural ideas and icons. This is so much the case that it is difficult to pierce through the cultural and ideological aura that surrounds these terms. To realistically reassess the meaning and function of autonomy in long-term care, then, requires that we pay attention to the symbolic meanings of autonomy and long-term care because these meanings not only set the context or stage for the analysis, but complicate its execution.

Long-Term Care Icons

The term *long-term care* conjures up many images, none of them felicitous. Long-term care hangs like a pall covering the inevitable coffin that awaits us all. Surprisingly, in our culture it is less death than long-term care that strikes us as so repugnant. This reaction may represent a psychological defense against death, to be sure, but its immediate effect is to place long-term care in an unfavorable light. The images of long-term care are images of frailty and despair, loneliness and destitution, and above all a profound sense of loss, a loss not only of things, but of who and what we are. These attitudes undoubtedly reflect society's perceptions of those institutions that are typically taken to be the central providers of long-term care, namely, nursing homes. These institutions have been portrayed in the media and described by anthropologists and sociologists as anything but humane (Gubrium 1975; Henry 1963; Kayser-Jones 1981; Laird 1979; Lidz, Fischer, and Arnold 1990; O'Brien 1989; Savishinsky 1991; Shield 1988; Vesperi 1983; Watson and Maxwell 1977).

Nursing homes are frequently seen as places of exploitation (of staff as well as residents), places that stimulate either moral outrage or revulsion that is captured in what surely must be a latent cultural icon—a blabbering, incoherent, disheveled elder strapped into a geri-chair beckoning or threatening some unseen others for help or warning and invariably ignored by staff who, without emotion, expression, or enthusiasm, mechanically carry on with the onerous tasks of daily bed and body work that is made even more difficult by the niggling demands of residents. The image is coupled with the olfactory assault of urine, excrement, and myriad other unpleasant odors that suffuses inevitably drab corridors or insipid sitting rooms where residents sit transfixed, each in their own world. There are also disturbing sounds of people moaning from down the hall, crying out, one elder scolding another harshly, others weeping in protest. No wonder that the pall of long-term care is feared as much as the coffin it covers! Long-term care seems suffused with a terrifying absence, the absence of any sense of control, dignity, or identity. It is a perverse state of living death, somewhere just this side of madness.

Like many cultural icons, the nursing home–dominated image of long-term care is in its general form brutally apt. Like all icons it also harbors latent meaning that requires careful exegesis and qualification. For one thing, not all long-term care is institutional. Statistics released in 1990 showed approximately 1,553,000 people residing in America's 25,646 nursing homes. The cost of their care came to $2.38 billion or 8.1 percent of the nation's total expenditure on health care. Seventy-nine percent of those individuals lived in privately owned institutions, 17 percent in voluntary, nonprofit institutions, and the remaining 4 percent in government-run facilities (U.S. Bureau of the Census 1990: 93, 104, 112).

Only 5 percent of those over age sixty-five were in long-term care on any given day, but of those in the sixty-five-plus age bracket in 1990, 43 percent will eventually reside for some period of time in a nursing home and two-thirds of them will be female. Twenty-five percent of those in institutions will spend at least twelve months there, while at least 10 percent will be patients for five years or more (Kemper and Murtaugh 1991: 597). The chances of being in a geriatric facility significantly increases with age. Approximately 22 percent of the elderly population will spend some time in one after they reach the age of 85 (Siegel and Taeuber 1986: 101). Most older people live outside nursing homes and in contact with their families and friends (Shanas 1979). Even for institutionalized elders, perhaps a score of individuals outside, such as family, friends, neighbors, clergy, social workers, lawyers, and doctors, will be involved in their care and directly touched by their fate (Savishinsky 1991: 9–10).

A considerable amount of care is thus delivered in the home either by family, friends, or in-home nursing services. Such care involves help with various tasks of daily living ranging from personal assistance and services such as food preparation, hygiene, administration of medication, to companionship, assistance in shopping, and entertainment. Indeed, discussions of long-term care frequently presume that the nursing home is the focus whereas in point of fact the nursing home must be seen as but one social response among many to what is itself a heterogeneous set of needs. Although the nursing home as an icon for long-term care is clearly misleading, its prominence indicates something quite significant about our latent cultural expectations and anxieties.

In reality there are, at least, two kinds of nursing homes (sometimes existing within the same physical structure): the so-called "skilled" nursing home and the institution that provides only "intermediate" care (Lidz, Fischer, and Arnold 1990). The distinction in kind makes an important practical difference. Medicare pays only for skilled nursing care, as does most private insurance. Medicare-paid nursing care is designed to aid the transition from hospital for elders who have suffered an acute health crisis. It is short term, rehabilitation-oriented. There are strict time, disease, and dollar limits. Although Medicare is the only real national long-term care program in existence at present, it is remarkably short-term oriented (Diamond 1986: 1288). Medicaid pays for nursing home care only after a patient has become indigent. As a social safety net, it is situated frightfully near the ground. No wonder elders (and their families) perceive its "support" with such apprehension, for it means a fall, sometimes a precipitously long fall, from economic sufficiency to indigence. This economic fact adds to the perception of long-term care as involving a loss of independence; for many elders in nursing home care, this is a simple, if hardly bearable, fact of everyday life. Elders declining in health and ability to care for themselves understandably live in apprehension of the economic (as well as psychological and social) consequences of their fall.

While Medicare and Medicaid are conceptually two different support systems for older people, they actually function sequentially: elders move from one to the other as they move toward becoming paupers (Diamond 1986: 1289). Elders do not really *receive* this public aid, rather they are *on* Medicaid. The distinction is not just grammatical. The state pays the nursing home, not the patient. Of the amount paid to the nursing home, the elder receives only a token from which all personal items must be paid. Destitution is clearly the norm for these individuals cut off from the discretionary income that in our society is the almost universal measure of social status and worth. This point applies equally to those who have recently fallen from economic grace, as well as to those who have always depended on public aid, because discretion over the use of even limited funds is as important for the poor as for the middle class or wealthy.

The everyday reality of the nursing home thus is strikingly dissonant with the popular image of retirement as a stable life full of activity and engagement. Despite the images of active retirement promoted by groups such as the American Association of Retired Persons (AARP), long-term care represents economical, psychological, and social instability. No wonder there is such a fascination with autonomy. It is a slogan for liberation of the frail and destitute old, though like many slogans it needs exegesis if it is to promote any practically effective and ethically defensible action. The symbolic meaning of the nursing home as an icon for long-term care can help us to understand both the attraction and limitation of the appeal to autonomy as a central ethical concern and principle for long-term care.

Given our revulsion at the sometimes brutal and stark reality of nursing home life, appealing to considerations of autonomy both salves our sense of moral outrage and yet preserves the distance that we so dearly want to maintain between ourselves and the sense of loss and incapacity that figuratively oozes from the image. Autonomy is attractive because it provides a ready-made vernacular of rights and obligations that seem to capture what at first glance bothers us about long-term care, namely, the effacement of autonomy, revealed in the pronounced dependence of nursing home existence.

Nursing homes are examples of what Erving Goffman termed *total institutions* (Goffman 1960; 1961). Like army barracks, mental hospitals, nunneries, or prisons, nursing homes are "total" in the sense that they completely isolate, control, and reconstitute the daily lives of their residents. This is accomplished by stripping away and reconstituting the identities of their residents through rituals of initiation and degradation and participation of the residents themselves in certain kinds of behaviors for gaining privileges or manipulating the system. Opposition to such institutions is a well-known theme in American social thought, though it should be pointed out that the consequences of the most enthusiastic criticism of such institutions, as in the case of the deinstitutionalization of the mentally ill, should give us serious pause. Panaceas, appealing as they seem in theory, seldom work in practice. In the case of severely debilitated elders, it is commonplace to acknowledge the need for institutional care, but to hope that these oppressive institutions are liberalized without examining the meaning and practical reality of liberalization too closely.

Figuring centrally in talk of liberalizing nursing home care is the concept of autonomy manifested in numerous well-intentioned proposals, such as insisting on full-disclosure preadmission agreements, creation of patient ombudsmen or nursing home ethics committees, or insisting on delineation and respect for a core or basic set of resident rights or establishment of detailed values histories for each resident (Hofland 1990). Collectively, these devices attend to what bothers us most about the surface reality of nursing home existence, yet saves us from having to deal with the messy deep reality of being old and frail, including the economic, physical, psychological, and social conditions that engender nursing home care and the more difficult ethical questions that it poses.

Autonomy

Like long-term care, autonomy involves a diffuse set of meanings. It would thus be a mistake to assume that autonomy has a consistent meaning or usage in either moral and political theory or practical and everyday contexts. Recent philosophical work on autonomy has included a discussion of a range of concerns that generally tends to avoid use of the term itself (Christman 1988; 1989). *Autonomy* refers to a broad set of qualities that are generally, though not universally, regarded with approval. Autonomy is taken to be equivalent to liberty, either positive or negative liberty in Isaiah Berlin's sense (1969: 118–72), self-rule, self-determination, freedom of will, dignity, integrity, individuality, independence, responsibility, and self-knowledge; it is also identified with the qualities of self-assertion, critical reflection, freedom from obligation, absence of external causation, and knowledge of one's own interest, and is related to actions, beliefs, reasons for acting, rules, the will of others, thoughts, as well as principles (Beauchamp and Childress 1983; Dworkin 1978; 1988). Treatment of autonomy in the gerontological literature has similarly noted a range of meanings (Thomasma 1984) involving a diverse set of tensions or polarities (Collopy 1986; 1988).

This wide range of usage suggests that it is unlikely that an essential or core meaning underlies these various employments; therefore, it would be futile to try to develop an essential definition of autonomy as a starting point for practical ethical analysis of long-term care. Rather than arguing for a precise core or essential definition of autonomy, it would be best to acknowledge that the meaning of autonomy is irremediably context-dependent. It would be wrong to conclude that these observations imply that the meaning of the concept is so relative that meaningful philosophical treatment is precluded. Certainly, some accounts of autonomy will fail—in part because they force the notion of autonomy to accomplish what it is incapable of achieving in certain contexts of inquiry—but other analyses will succeed contextually. The important point is that philosophical treatments of autonomy must come to terms with the contextual nature of its meaning instead of relying on abstract, theoretically provided definitions.

Autonomy, however, is not only an important philosophical concept, but a significant cultural ideal. In the guise of independence, it has been a perennial feature of American society. In the early days of the Republic, Alexis de Tocqueville noted the peculiar tendency of Americans to draw apart and to keep to themselves: "Each citizen is disposed to isolate himself from the mass of his fellows and to draw apart with his family and friends. It not only makes each man forget his forefathers, but it conceals him from his descendants and separates him from his contemporaries" (quoted in Christiansen 1983: 35). More recently, American society has been characterized as "the lonely crowd" (Riesman 1950) and as engaged in a collective "pursuit of loneliness" (Slater 1970). Indeed, some authors have noted that the concept of individual freedom held by elderly Americans and their families rests on a sweeping faith and confidence of the individual in his own competence and mastery which, in turn, produces a definition of personal identity predicated on independence and self-reliance (Clark 1971: 265). This cultural ideal results in a variety of secondary defenses against dependence: a denial of need, hostility toward helpers even in the face of disabilities and limitations that require assistance from others, contempt for the real or imagined weakness of others, and, in some cases, an inflated self-image. The cultural attitude that constitutes an aversion for dependence has been termed *counterdependence* (Christiansen 1983: 52–128; Rogers 1974).

The attitude of counterdependence assumes that any form of dependence is tantamount to a degrading submission. This view is understandable given the dominance of the concept of autonomy as negative freedom, namely, the idea that individual freedom consists fundamentally in the noninterference of others in the life of the individual. The overdetermination of negative freedom is partly due to its association in Anglo-American political and ethical theory with a set of beliefs about individual freedom that prominently include self-reliance, personal preference, and self-assertion. (Christiansen 1983: 41–44)

Self-reliance refers to the capacity to provide for one's own needs. In the course of aging, however, dependence begins as the diminishment of one's powers of self-reliance. The problem is not with self-reliance as such, but rather that self-reliance defines individual worth. Lacking the ability to be self-reliant contributes to the feeling of worthlessness experienced by many old people. If identity and value are grounded in one's ability to be self-supporting, then physical infirmity and disability can compromise one's sense of personal worth precisely through compromising self-reliance. This point is admirably summarized in the notion of "active life expectancy" as an empirical measure of population health. This measure involves activities and abilities such as bathing, dressing, transfer or mobility, and eating that are correlated with a sense of functional well-being; loss of these functional abilities represents loss of independence (Katz, Branch, *et al.* 1983).

A second concept associated with the idea of individual freedom is personal preference. Personal preference focuses discussion of autonomy on the phenomena of choice and decision. Indeed, choice is of such importance that attention to one's wishes, desires, and impulses comprise a significant set of concerns in the ethical analysis of human action. This focus, however, makes it difficult, if not impossible, to question whether the values implied by one's desires, impulses, or wishes are worth having. From the fact that I choose something on the basis of my desire, for example, a certain kind of food, it does not follow that that something is good for me. Attention to my wants or preferences, however, not only renders the question of the good of the objects of choice irrelevant, it restricts the domain of ethics to but one feature among many defining human moral agency. Choice is undeniably important, but not all-important. Attention to the phenomena of choice and decisionmaking has had the unfortunate consequence of rendering otiose other features of autonomy.

Third, the concept of individual freedom includes the value of self-assertion as a basic requirement, namely, that one actively pursue the fulfillment of one's desires. It is not enough to have desires or to make choices; one must be actively engaged in their fulfillment or accomplishment. So construed, autonomy commits individuals to a seeming ceaseless pursuit of the fulfillment of their preferences, for without such fulfillment autonomy itself is seen as useless or empty. Whatever thwarts the attainment of one's desires is seen as curtailing freedom; hence, noninterference becomes the obvious imperative under this concept of autonomy. It is commonly admitted, however, that this view is odd and even destructive when applied to children, yet the restraint or mastery of desire that is necessary for, indeed, one might say definitive of, maturation seems to be thought of as somehow inappropriate or wrong in the case of adults! A moment's reflection should indicate that this is a fundamental mistake. Acquiring any sort of skill or expertise, whether as a child or adult, involves discipline of unruly tendencies or desires. Learning always involves a subordination of the immediate fulfillment of desire to wider ends and purposes.

Autonomy and Long-Term Care: The Problem

The dissonance between the image of the robust, striving, and unencumbered individual making her own way competently in the world and even the most banal limitations that underlie the need for long-term care should be readily apparent. Some adult individuals, for example, frail elders, are generally not fully self-reliant; they often lack the psychological ability, physical energy, or social and economic prerequisites necessary to pursue their preferences. The view of autonomy that takes as a defining feature the pursuit of *all* preferences—just because those preferences are preferences of the individual—seems to foredoom as paternalistic and objectionable any attempt to respond to an elder's evident need. Where desire reigns, need recedes. Thus, the diminished capacity that brings elders into long-term care contributes to the view that dependence entails subservience and inferiority; but if independence is only, or primarily, valued, then we should not be surprised to find that responding even to basic human needs is fraught with contradiction.

Addressing the conjunction of autonomy and long-term care thus presents two types of problems at two different levels: first, the level of concepts involving the meaning of long-term care and the meaning of autonomy and, second, the practical difficulties associated with actual autonomy and the reality of long-term care. These four elements interplay in a complex pattern. For ease of analysis, I take up these elements in a way that unavoidably introduces a degree of abstraction that runs counter to the main thesis of this work, namely, that autonomy in long-term care should be approached in a phenomenologically concrete fashion. I simply do not see how I could have done otherwise.

The most striking feature of long-term care is that adult individuals suffering from diseases and illnesses of being old experience a compromised vigor and ability to function that requires regular care ranging from help in the activities of daily living, such as housework, food preparation, and hygiene, to highly skilled nursing and medical care. Elders requiring long-term care are, as a class, defined by functional disabilities that frequently bring with them vulnerabilities as well. Because elders requiring long-term care often deviate in obvious ways from the ideal of the competent, rational, and free decision maker that is implicit in the commonplace understanding of autonomy, various mechanisms have been devised to protect elders from unwarranted intrusion. These mechanisms include the use of various legal advocacy and guardianship measures to endow elders with specific rights as well as the use of surrogate decision-making procedures, especially in the case of refusal of life-sustaining medical care. Reliance on surrogate decision-making is an interesting development in long-term care, primarily growing out of the acute care context (Buchanan and Brock 1989). The reality of long-term care apparently forces even the staunchest proponent of autonomy as independence to deal with the reality of an impaired decision-making capacity or incompetence that is an ineliminable feature of long-term care.

This response is both understandable and troubling. It is understandable because the reality is such that elderly individuals who require long-term care frequently experience various physical, psychological, and social disabilities and deprivations that should give us pause. These frailties suggest that the ideal of the person that underlies the standard view of autonomy is inapplicable in many of these cases or simply fails to provide much practical assistance for either restoring or sustaining the degree and kind of autonomy that is present. Primarily because it is dominated by an abstract and ideal concept of the autonomous individual that fails to jibe with the reality of long-term care, the concept of autonomy as independence simply proves inadequate and has to be refurbished if it is to function importantly in the context of long-term care.

These observations point to the second problem that arises if we critically reflect on the applicability and usefulness of commonplace understandings of autonomy in long-term care, namely, the nature of autonomy itself. The traditional liberal view of autonomy tends to direct attention to specific problems associated with decisionmaking. This view is not surprising given the powerful place that the related concepts of independence, self-determination, and rights enjoy in our culture. These concepts, embodied in the Anglo-American legal system, exert a significant influence on bioethical thinking. Hence, autonomy has come to be defined primarily in terms of a concept of human persons as rational, independent agents and decision makers, who are assumed to be competent and who can be understood without serious reference to society or history.

Independent decision makers are insulated by a fabric of rights that protect them from the intrusive and coercive influence of the state or other individuals. Indeed, the individual is often seen as standing in opposition to society or the state that is assumed to pose a threat to the integrity of the self. Individuals are idealized in such a way that the expression of uniquely individual beliefs and values is given primacy over other goods or values. Furthermore, decisionmaking is regarded as a rational process that can be understood or explained in terms of decision theory; communicative interactions between individuals are thought to involve primarily the exchange of information as evidenced by the stress on disclosure of information in the legal doctrine of informed consent. This view of autonomy is remarkably abstract and assumes an ideal view of persons. It is not only deficient as a general theory of the meaning of actual autonomy, but, more pointedly, is not well suited for conceptualizing the ethical problems associated with long-term care. For this reason, the concept of autonomy itself must be reassessed and revamped if it is to play a significant role in theoretically and practically clarifying the ethics of long-term care.

The assumptions and implications of the commonplace understanding of autonomy as independence orient reflection on long-term care to relatively dramatic conflicts expressible in terms of rights. As a consequence, more mundane day-to-day experiences and encounters of elders with caregivers in long-term care tend to be overlooked, in part, because they lack the conflictual, dramatic, and discrete characteristics required by the standard view. A truly helpful ethics of long-term care, however, would incorporate a concept of autonomy that is interstitial to the typical everyday reality of long-term care, not one that fixates on the unusual or atypical. The context from which the main concept of autonomy comes is the political/legal realm; it is further supported by the reality of acute care medicine that hand-in-glove seems to support a concept of ethics that is problem or issue based. Unfortunately, it also tends to be insensitive to questions of responsibility, quality of care, and the affective dimension of clinical encounters, concerns that are significant in long-term care as well.

The common view that autonomy is tantamount to independence has important implications for long-term care. First, the cultural dominance of this model of autonomy creates a backlash against dependence of any sort, so that the frail and infirm old who require long-term care are especially vulnerable to the pejorative meanings associated with dependence. They are seen and frequently see themselves as burdensome and less than full persons. As a class these elders are treated as deviants from the images of robustly active retirement cultivated by groups such as the American Association of Retired Persons (AARP) for which the oxymoron *active retirement* has become a battle cry.

Second, autonomy as independence injects a predominantly adversarial and conflictual set of metaphors into thinking about long-term care. Like so much discourse in our society, the language of rights eclipses other ethical language. As a result, long-term care is mainly thought of in terms of problems that can or should be secured by establishing legal rights or promulgating regulations. The goal of these efforts is to force caregivers to conform to the standards of a liberal polity and respect the rights of their wards. Ironically, when elders lose the abilities assumed to be present for autonomy as independence, society is less enthusiastically committed to dealing with the aftermath. Frail and sick elders are infantilized by social institutions and programs like Medicare and Medicaid that afford elders entitlements to *services*, but synergistically impose destitution and isolation on those requiring nursing and other supportive *care*.

Third, the asymmetry between autonomy as negative freedom (the vision of the agent as independent and rationally competent) and the economic, physical, psychological, and social needs of elders propelled into long-term care forces to prominence the question "Is autonomy really the central value and concept for thinking about the ethics of long-term care?" I clearly think that it is, but only after it is revised can it provide an ethically robust framework for the practice of long-term care.

The goal of this work is to articulate just such a framework without completely rejecting the central commitments of the liberal view of autonomy. I propose a complementary framework to open the everyday reality of long-term care to ethical analysis. This alternative framework develops a view of the nature of actual autonomy predicated on a concrete understanding of the everyday experience of long-term care. This framework involves a shift of attention from autonomy as independence to actual autonomy as it appears in the everyday world of life by articulating a developmentally oriented and phenomenologically adequate account of autonomy in terms of concrete human action in the social world. By bringing into focus the full range of caregiving interactions as well as the structure of caregiving relationships, this account opens up the complex reality of the long-term care of elders for clinical ethical reflection.

2

The Liberal Theory of Autonomy

Autonomy has become a touchstone for much analysis and discussion in medical ethics. To understand its scope in the context of long-term care, it is important to appreciate the lineage and limitations of this concept in the liberal theory of autonomy. Although there are significant problems associated with this view of autonomy, these problems are tractable. I argue that liberal theory need not be rejected, but rather confined within its proper borders and supplemented in ethical analysis and practice by a fuller and more adequate view of what it means to be an autonomous agent in the world. My discussion of these points is thus part of a wider debate over the modern, liberal view of the self and the political and ethical commitments of this view. I provide only marginal reference to this debate, mainly as it bears on the more limited concern of this work.

I argue that liberal theory affords an inadequate vantage point from which to survey the ethics of providing long-term care for impaired elders, but want to avoid a position that simply displaces autonomy in favor of other principles or values, for example, community, tradition, or beneficence. These values do have a place in my account, but as aspects of a fuller understanding of the meaning of human autonomy.

Although I take the liberal theory of autonomy seriously, I argue that it should be restricted to the political/legal realm. This restriction clears the field for developing an alternative treatment of autonomy in subsequent chapters. In the course of the present chapter, I discuss the communitarian critique of liberalism and argue that both views share suspect assumptions about the nature of justification in ethics. I defend a contextualist alternative which has practical implications for the analysis of autonomy in the context of long-term care. Finally, I argue that rights language does play an important, but circumscribed role in long-term care and that a parentalist approach to caring for frail and dependent elders needs to be distinguished from paternalism, the liberal bête noire.

Pluralism, Toleration, and Neutrality

Autonomy is a central value in American society; it gives expression to a broad set of legal and political ideals that have gone under the name of liberalism. Central to political liberalism is the idea of individual freedom or autonomy. As a term *autonomy* refers to a broad set of qualities that are generally, though not universally, regarded with approval in our society. Central to its treatment in political contexts is the concept of independence or what has been termed *negative freedom*, the freedom to be left alone (Berlin 1969). Implicit in this negative concept, to be sure, is a positive concept involving qualities of self-assertion, critical reflection, absence of external causation, and knowledge of one's own interest, qualities that are themselves indeterminately related to concepts of actions, beliefs, and reasons for acting (Dworkin 1988). The mainstream treatments of autonomy, however, usually have little to say about the positive characteristics or capacities that are required for negative freedom and are content instead to worry about the kind of social arrangements that interfere with the exercise of individual freedom of action or choice (Young 1986). These treatments are expressive of deep-seated cultural values that comprise the conceptual context for my examination of autonomy and long-term care.

As a cultural ideal, autonomy usually involves a vision of individuals freely living their lives according to their own beliefs and values with minimal interference by the state or others. Minimal involvement or intrusion of the state is permitted, for example, to regulate and secure public safety because of the belief that such involvement ultimately promotes or permits individual freedom of action and choice. In things that matter most, however, other individuals and the state should have no say. Indeed, implicit in the cultural value of autonomy is a deep suspicion about shared beliefs and values. Things are essentially valuable because they are valued by autonomous individuals. Along with skepticism about external authority is a deep-seated relativism about values and the moral good.

Given the stress on individuality and skepticism about beliefs and values that do not happen to be *one's own*—I leave the meaning of this crucial phrase unexamined as it typically is in the context under discussion—proponents of the liberal theory defend two further concepts, namely, pluralism and toleration, as unavoidable corollaries of autonomy. *Pluralism* is the view that there are many viable concepts of the good life, many viable concepts of how one's life should be conducted. These concepts are neither different versions of a single homogeneous good nor related in any discernible hierarchical pattern. Thus, difference is unavoidable and ineliminable. As a result of difference, conflicts and disagreement unavoidably arise in the course of daily living. For this reason, toleration is an essential corollary of pluralism. Because we can expect that even reasonable persons will disagree about fundamental values and concepts of the good life, practical acceptance of the views of others—views that we may find wrongheaded, objectionable, or even repulsive—is required. Since liberals accept that we must live with those who do not share our own ideals or else succumb to interminable conflict or resort to force to settle disagreement, toleration is the logical requirement.

Given that diversity of viewpoints (pluralism) and disagreement among reasonable persons have become features of modern life and medical practice, political liberalism is the doctrine that the state should be neutral with respect to such disputes. An action or decision will count as neutral only if its justification does not appeal to some presumed intrinsic superiority of its own concept of the good life. Neutrality understood in this procedural fashion thus is silent on the specific goals that the liberal society ought to pursue; this does not necessarily mean that neutrality requires a so-called minimal state, that is, a state that, for the most part, renounces substantive commitments that embody the content of any particular vision of the good, even though libertarians frequently assume just such a conclusion (Nozick 1974).

Liberals need not deny that freedom could or should mean more than the absence of governmental interference in nonpolitical areas (Larmore 1987: 47). So it would be consistent, though rare, for an avowed liberal to defend substantive ideals of (positive) freedom, including, for example, ideals of self-realization or the provision of "meaningful" choices. These positive ideals, however, could be defended on ethical grounds. Because political neutrality need not be absolute, other substantive moral commitments are possible, even required, on a liberal perspective. Indeed, the liberal advocacy of negative freedom occurs most forcefully when particular ideas of the good life or ideals of *positive* autonomy are pressed on unwilling or unwitting persons in the public and political realm. The rights to informed consent and treatment refusal, are well-known examples of the application of the principle of noninterference to health care. Such rights protect vulnerable patients from the authority and power of health professionals and institutions alike.

The ideal of neutrality requires that the state should not promote any particular concept of the good life because of its presumed "intrinsic" superiority. It is important to note that this neutrality is not a neutrality of outcome but procedure. Some visions of the good life may in fact be supported and, indeed, flourish under a liberal state, though others will not. For example, ideals of the good life that are open in principle to everyone, whatever one's cultural or religious background, may well be stronger under a liberal state than are sectarian views that are exclusionary. Exclusionary views do not flourish in a liberal state not because the liberal state cannot support the *content* of their ideals, but because the liberal state *procedurally* restrains sectarian forces to prevent a political imposition of particular points of view (Larmore 1987: 44).

Such a view comprises what Charles Larmore aptly termed a *modus vivendi*. So regarded, neutrality is simply a means of accommodation (Larmore 1987: 74). It is a position that is adopted to solve specific political problems that arise out of the conflict between various commitments that people have. It is *not* a substantive position that expresses a full moral theory of final purposes and values. Neutrality constitutes a modus vivendi between persons whose ultimate ideals are—or could be—either incompatible or fundamentally in conflict; as such, its very existence assumes that other substantive ideals exist independently and are consistently seen to exist outside liberal theory. Autonomy understood as negative freedom thus represents a political commitment, an ideal that regulates public interactions, but not necessarily a substantive component of the moral life. The modus vivendi view of political neutrality accepts that substantive views of what constitutes the good exist outside the political realm. This view of neutrality and the meaning of autonomy differs importantly from its opposite, the expressivist perspective.

The *expressivist perspective* understands political neutrality as the expression of a fundamental kind of detachment that humans should have if they are to flourish. The neutrality of the liberal state on this view is thus not simply a corollary of autonomy understood as negative freedom in the realm of politics, but as the highest *personal* ideal. On this interpretation, independence and distance from particular substantive commitments, goals, or values underpins, indeed justifies, the neutrality characteristic of the liberal state. Clearly, the expressivist defense of negative freedom relies on a positive account of the nature of the autonomous subject. Some authors have argued that the main problem with this view is that the concept of personal autonomy is derived from political theory as if politics defined the core sense of the person or self. The positive model of the self defended by expressivists is remarkably consonant with the self as conceived in political theory, but it is a mistake to attribute to political theory alone the deficiencies of the expressivist view of the self as fundamentally detached. The sources of this account are much more diverse. Nonetheless, at bottom, this account of the nature of the self abstracts even from commonsensical understandings of what it means to be a person as an agent in the world. Whether this abstraction is ultimately motivated by political theory, a misguided ethical theory, or other considerations is a question that need not detain us. The implication of this perspective, whatever its origin, is important because it affords an extremely thin and morally deficient vision of what it is to be a person needing long-term care. Whatever its theoretical roots, this point of view seems to express cultural attitudes about the person as an agent that will repay further analysis in subsequent chapters.

There are, to be sure, other reasons to question, if not reject, the expressivist account (Larmore 1987; Young 1986). The standard criticisms of the extension of negative freedom to the whole of morality are typically based on a wide-ranging argument about the nature of morality and politics. Although I draw on these wider discussions, I reference them only to the extent that they helpfully apply to the special problem of conceptualizing autonomy in the context of long-term care. The expressivist and modus vivendi perspectives provide competing views of the nature of the state in supporting particular belief systems. Acceptance of the modus vivendi position keeps the main themes of liberal theory intact without (the expressivist) commitment to a view of the self and the good life dependent ultimately on autonomy as negative freedom. Positive accounts of autonomy are still possible, though such accounts will necessarily be ethical and not political in intent.

On this view of liberal theory, then, neutrality is basically a *political* ideal. Individual freedom is protected by the state procedurally by political and legal mechanisms to allow private relations to develop without constraint. For this reason, political freedom is a relatively restricted concept. It covers only the right of the person not to be unjustifiably interfered with by the state. This negative concept has a positive component as well that is sometimes overlooked in libertarian positions: the state is not only constrained not to act, but also obligated to assure that others (e.g., individuals or groups) also respect this right of individuals to be left alone. Hence, the negative freedom to be left alone frequently requires more than mere forbearance on the part of the state; it requires the enforcement of this right for its citizens.

Costs are always associated with the enforcement or protection of this right to negative freedom. Thus, negative or liberty rights are not "free" as is sometimes claimed; ideally only forbearance is strictly required, but practically more than forbearance is involved. Protection of liberty entails costs that themselves involve restrictions of liberty (e.g., to assure public safety and protection of rights by police requires payment that depends on taxation). Even in Isaiah Berlin's classic treatment (1969: 118–62), negative liberty is a political ideal that need not exhaust everything that is meant by the term *freedom*.

Ronald Dworkin's critique of negative freedom is particularly pertinent (1977). Dworkin argues that there is no general right to liberty, but only rights to specific liberties that are compatible with the equality of concern and respect for all. Liberties are thus grounded in terms of the fundamental equality of persons, not in a view of the self as irremediably individual and isolated. The fundamental principle is thus a relational one, not just in the formal sense that equality is a principle that is applied to all persons, but substantively in that both concern and respect constitute responses to other persons (Christiansen 1983: 158)

Dworkin's argument also pairs respect with concern. Respect for persons has been interpreted by many thinkers as nothing more than forbearance, namely, respecting a person's negative right to noninterference. Dworkin argues that respect involves treating others as "human beings who are capable of forming and acting on intelligent conceptions of how their lives should be lived" and concern involves treating others as "human beings who are capable of suffering and frustration" (Dworkin 1977: 278). As a fundamental ethical attitude, concern requires that people be alert to the deprivation of others and be ready and available to relieve their suffering whenever that is possible. In the absence of clear cases of suffering and deprivation, the principle of respect requires deference to the capacity of human persons for forming and acting on intelligent conceptions of how their lives should be lived. Dworkin's analysis thus provides an important place for concern alongside respect for autonomy in an account of rights founded not on negative freedom, but a principle of equality.

Some writers have questioned the distinction between negative and positive notions of liberty (Feinberg 1973; MacCallum 1967) arguing that they cannot be analyzed independently, though the tendency of many thinkers is to do just that. In what should the positive ideals of freedom consist is certainly a matter of dispute, but it should not be forgotten that in the liberal view government is precluded from imposing any one candidate over all others. This does not end the discussion, but simply points to the limitations of the question as it is posed politically. Instead, the issue is marked out as properly a matter of ethics, not a matter to be resolved politically through the public imposition of law.

The important feature of neutrality for present purposes is that it is a uniquely *political* ideal. It governs the public relations between persons and the state, not the private relations between persons or between persons and other institutions.

Negative freedom, the freedom to be left alone to pursue one's own choices, is also a uniquely political ideal. This political ideal, however, does seem to be the model for our society's understanding of individual autonomy. The autonomous state is characterized by independence from the laws and governance of other states. To be autonomous in this sense, then, is to be sovereign or to have an unfettered authority within a specific political domain, no matter what other conditions prevail (Young 1986: 7).

Influenced by this ideal, individual autonomy is regarded analogously as involving independence from the authority of others—state, institutions, or other individuals. Autonomy so regarded has obvious affinities with the concept of negative liberty articulated by Isaiah Berlin (1969: 122), namely, that to be at liberty is to be unobstructed by others, as well as with those accounts of rights as defining spheres of activities in which interference by others is illegitimate (Richards 1981; Wellman 1985: 102). Most versions of the political model, however, contain a serious deficiency, namely, the failure to account for the fact that various conditions, such as economic underdevelopment, can make it impossible for states to control their own destinies in meaningful ways even though they continue to make and administer their own laws (Young 1986: 7). Thus, even at the level of the state, the model is somewhat simplistic.

Economic conditions (among others) also severely restrict the options open to individuals and so restrict their liberty in important ways (Feinberg 1978). Such restrictions seem an essential fact of life, and so are unavoidable aspects of autonomy; but, they are seldom given serious attention by liberal theorists. There are many reasons for this omission, but they share the common feature that liberal accounts typically operate at a level of abstraction that is far removed from actual empirical reality. This abstract orientation creates special problems for long-term care because the everyday detail of actual cases and circumstances of autonomy tend to get washed out. To reassess autonomy in long-term care requires that a positive account of autonomy be developed to restore the lost concreteness. For the moment, it is important to be clear how liberal theory typically understands the relationship of the state and positive expressions of autonomy.

The distinction between the public and the private employed in the above analysis is likely to prove troublesome for some. Surely, one might argue, a significant amount of institutional long-term care is public, not private. It is public in the sense that it is funded with government monies. Analogously, one might even insist that some home care is public in that the source of funding and regulations ensure that the state is always nearby to scrutinize interactions between professional care providers and clients. These observations are true enough, but the distinction between the public and the private goes deeper. The public realm is properly regarded as that social realm in which individuals are regarded as strangers. Individuals are treated in terms of the minimal demands of morality. That is why the language of autonomy in the political/legal realm is so important and finds expression in terms of various rights and corresponding obligations. Such rights protect individuals by defining noninterference as a primary principle regulating interactions. In caregiving situations, however, noninterference as a primary ethical principle makes very little sense.

Care involves varying degrees of intimacy and affective interaction, interaction that cannot be regulated by a principle that inflexibly pits caregiver and client against one another. (I discuss this point further in the section "Nursing Home Admission Practices.") Hence, a concern to enhance and protect the autonomy of elders in such circumstances must turn from politically and legally motivated articulations of autonomy toward other models for guidance.

The State and Positive Autonomy

The role of the state, according to liberal theory, primarily should be to enhance the ability of individuals to freely pursue their own life-style and preferences. Liberal theory thus strongly supports the right of elders—as well as other competent adults—to decide what constitutes their own best interests. This theory extends even to the point of supporting the right of individuals to refuse life-sustaining treatment. For the most part, the freedoms defended by liberal theory are negative, namely, freedom from the interference of others. As discussed earlier, it is commonly, though mistakenly, assumed—for example, by libertarians—that a liberal state is prevented from defining positive rights or entitlements since providing such rights necessarily entails the restriction of other freedoms because such rights inevitably have costs associated with them. A minimal state that guaranteed only procedural rights supporting independence is not necessarily required by liberal theory. Other more ample versions of the state and its role in defining positive rights are also defensible on liberal grounds. For example, although individuals are free to choose what is in their best interest, it may be necessary for the state to provide services that instrumentally enable individuals to pursue their vision of the good life. Assuring fair access to a basic minimum of health care is one example in which a liberal state could legitimately structure social institutions to achieve positive outcomes (Agich 1991; Buchanan 1991; Daniels 1985; 1988; President's Commission 1983).

In the case of long-term care, the services provided might be predicated on the recognition that suffering from disabling conditions in old age itself thwarts autonomy. These supports, however, should be compatible with a variety of normative moral beliefs and commitments. They should, in other words, be nonsectarian and should enable individuals, insofar as practically possible, to exercise their independent choices or to live out their old age in terms of their own value commitments and beliefs. Thus, elders not only enjoy liberal rights to noninterference, including rights to informed consent and treatment refusal, but more important liberal theory is compatible with social and medical support systems for elders, even though salient problems, such as intergenerational justice and the moral claim to resources, need to be resolved (Callahan 1985, 1987; Daniels 1988). Substantively expansive visions of the state, therefore, are not prohibited by liberal theory for logical reasons, though widely shared assumptions about the nature of the liberal state historically influenced many thinkers to conclude just the opposite.

The evolution of the idea of a neutral state was influenced historically as much by beliefs that the free market was the most effective way to produce and distribute wealth and resources as by any logical requirements of liberal political theory itself. The conditions of a free market and the requirements of a liberal state became affiliated to such an extent that they are frequently taken to be one and the same, though nothing in liberal theory specifically requires the existence of free market conditions. Indeed, one might cynically point out the rhetoric of the free market frequently is used to oppose egalitarian or redistributivist programs for the less fortunate such as welfare, but not government programs such as import restrictions that help special interests. Thinking that political neutrality logically entails a free market, and by implication excludes all state involvement, shows the extent to which neutrality is seen as a substantive, rather than a procedural requirement. Expressivist positions are especially prone to this mistake.

A liberal state, especially with the modus vivendi view, is not logically precluded from actively structuring social institutions, including the market, to achieve ends justified on liberal grounds. Although individuals are free to decide what is in their best interest, it may be necessary for the state to provide some set of basic services in order to enable individuals to pursue their own vision of the good life. Assuring fair access to education, employment, health care, and housing are areas in which a liberal state could legitimately structure social institutions to achieve substantive outcomes. Health care is thus one among many such areas. In fact, the role of the state in the regulation of certain aspects of long-term care is already quite evident. Rather than considering such regulation as intrusive on theoretical grounds, it is better to ask whether the regulations in place achieve the kind of outcomes that a liberal state *should* support. To answer this question adequately, a positive account of the meaning of autonomy in long-term care is necessary. Before such an account can be developed, it is important to be clear why liberal thinkers have reservations about positive accounts of autonomy.

Some Problems of Positive Autonomy

Many liberal thinkers give primacy to negative liberty, indeed, even to the point of rejecting positive concepts of liberty as inevitably involving a totalitarian or authoritarian stance (Berlin 1969: 131). It is also sometimes said in defense of the primacy of autonomy conceived as negative liberty that positive views of autonomy necessarily entail an unjustified commitment to a metaphysical postulate regarding a real or higher self, what Isaiah Berlin termed, *the inner citadel* (1969: 135–41); so that to speak of positive autonomy requires that one differentiate a real or essential self from superficial or phenomenal expressions (Young 1986: 5). Others, however, have trenchantly argued that the liberal suspicion and criticism of positive autonomy, based both on its fear of the alleged authoritarian or totalitarian implications of treatments of positive autonomy and its claim that positive autonomy involves an unjustified metaphysical commitment regarding self, are largely unjustified (Larmore 1987; Young 1986). I, too, believe that liberal suspicion and criticism of positive autonomy are not fully justified. Nothing in liberal theory logically precludes positive treatments of autonomy, though many versions of liberal theory do in fact harbor serious reservations about positive accounts. The specific concerns about authoritarian and metaphysical commitments in positive accounts of autonomy merit further discussion, particularly in the context of long-term care.

First, the alleged authoritarian—more commonly regarded as paternalistic—dangers of positive autonomy, though relevant, need to be balanced by the requirement of concern for frail elders. Simply to rely on the accepted understanding of autonomy as independence without inquiring into its meaning and significance for a frail or disabled elder demonstrates a questionable apathy or insincerity at best. Such attitudes need to be set aside if the question of the ethics of long-term care is to be the subject of serious attention. Nonetheless, there is good reason to accept the (limited) relevance of traditional worries about authoritarian impulses nestled in the language of positive accounts of autonomy and its values. For one thing, practices such as the widespread use of restraints on confused, cognitively impaired, or wandering elders for the sake of prevention of injury need serious rebuttal. One obvious way to do so is by attacking the authoritarian or paternalistic stance of the "protectors" of the safety of these elders.

Second, the suspicions of suppressed metaphysical commitments regarding higher senses of self are not rarified philosophical or theoretical concerns, but bear directly on the practical reality of long-term care. Elders requiring long-term care suffer from many disabling conditions, including severe ones such as dementia, that call into question the applicability of any normative standard that involves reference to a "higher" self. Does the *higher self* refer to an actual or ideal entity, a past or present entity or state? If positive accounts of autonomy require a view of an intact self, how could they helpfully clarify cases of dementia or severe confusion? These are not insignificant questions. Worries about paternalism and metaphysical commitments are serious enough to merit attention in any account that is broadly liberal and that purports a positive vision of actual autonomy, and so they are especially pertinent for assessing autonomy in the context of long-term care. Both the limitations and positive implications of the liberal model of autonomy for long-term care thus require further exploration.

Liberal thought is an expression of fundamental cultural attitudes regarding not only autonomy, but what it means to be a person and the nature of value, that cannot be lightly dismissed. Autonomy has become a core concept of medical ethics. The liberal treatment of autonomy is important for long-term care if its preoccupation with negative freedom is seen as a component of a justifiable, or at least plausible, political theory, but nothing more. The liberal defense of autonomy as negative freedom, in other words, is restricted to the realm of politics and law leaving open the analysis of concepts of positive autonomy to ethics without the need for further apology. This strategy has been admirably developed in Charles Larmore's (1987) argument that liberal theory is primarily a political, not an ethical theory. When properly confined to the realm of politics and law, liberal principles are both plausible and defensible. The unbridled extension into the realm of ethics, however, leads to unsatisfactory, even repugnant, outcomes. The challenge for a positive account of autonomy in long-term care is to develop an ethical framework that supplements, rather than completely rejects, the liberal view.

Liberal Principles in Long-Term Care

Despite their limitations, liberal ideas have important implications for long-term care. The liberal version of autonomy provides a historically important foundation for the establishment of certain rights to information, privacy, and so on that are as important in long-term care as in other contexts of health care and social life. Such rights globally serve to assure that elders are not forced to adopt visions of the good life that are not their own. In their most general form, these are rights to be left alone. In ethical terms, these rights remind us that nonmaleficence is more important as a principle of action than beneficence, that is, not harming individuals as they would judge harm is more important than pursuing a particular "good" for individuals that they themselves would refuse to acknowledge or accept as good. Although these advantages are well recognized, they have untoward side effects in long-term care, some of which parallel those evident in other contexts of health care.

Liberal principles seem to imply that individuals have what has been termed in the psychiatric context a "right to rot" (Appelbaum and Gutheil 1979; Gutheil and Appelbaum 1980). The liberty principle is taken as so fundamental that the right to be left alone is maintained no matter what the actual condition of the individual is and no matter what harm results. Such a "right" would support the abandonment of elders to their illnesses, disabilities, and distress. It would provide a general basis for ignoring the plight of helpless individuals. One could thus insist on the right of elders to be left alone in the name of autonomy, when interventions, such as providing transportation, actually expand the range of action and choice of elders. Such an outcome is highly undesirable and, indeed, ethically repugnant. For this reason, many have tried to argue generally against liberalism and the liberal ideals of pluralism and toleration by insisting that communitarian or other nonneutral concepts of the good life can serve to justify interference. This move is basically mistaken, since the real problem is the unbridled scope accorded the specific principle of negative freedom rather than the broad liberal view in which neutrality and toleration are understood to be limited *political* principles.

The liberal view of autonomy does provide a broad political and legal framework by which the state ensures that elders shall not be discriminated against and that they shall be protected from the unwanted intrusions of others. That implication is generally defensible; it provides the theoretical foundation for the principles of informed consent and respect for patients that are salutary developments in medical ethics. Generally, the creation and implementation of patient rights is a positive outcome that is admirably defended in terms of the liberal principle of autonomy, though it should be acknowledged that confining discussion to such rights does raise dilemmas such as the problem of determining competence (Macklin 1983a; 1983b), a matter that standard accounts of autonomy usually finesse. Two examples readily illustrate the relevance of autonomy as negative freedom to long-term care: nursing home admission practices and the use of physical and other restraints.

Nursing Home Admission Practices

Whatever the reasons, nursing home admissions frequently occur under stress and in circumstances of crisis. No matter how wrong the choice turns out to be, it is frequently final because of "transfer trauma" and inertia (Taylor 1981). In many places, elders' choice is limited by the availability of nursing home beds and by the unwillingness of many nursing homes to accept Medicaid patients. Typically, elders themselves are seldom actively involved in the admissions process. Even when clearly competent, elders are frequently not asked to sign their own admission contract (Ambrogi and Gerard 1986; Buckingham 1987). Investigation of nursing home admission contracts has concluded that they typically contain unlawfully restrictive contract language and that elders and their representatives are rarely fully aware of its content or implications of the agreement that they sign (Ambrogi 1990; Ambrogi and Gerard 1986; Ambrogi and Leonard 1988a; 1988b; Legal Services for the Elderly 1983; Schneider and Oliver 1987; Subcommittee on Law and the Elderly 1987).

Virtually all nursing home admission agreements are adhesion contracts, standardized form contracts that are characterized by unequal power relations (Ambrogi 1990: 73). Although theoretically subject to negotiation, these contracts are usually offered on a take-it or leave-it basis. Many contracts misrepresent the extent of the institution's liability under the law. They contain exculpatory clauses or waivers of liability that seek to limit liability or excuse the institution altogether for the negligence of its staff or attending physicians, for injury caused to a resident by another resident or by wandering away from the institution, for theft or loss of personal property, and for injury or damage caused by smoking. The effect of this misrepresentation is to intimidate and discourage elders from pursuing valid claims (Brown 1985; Nemore 1985). Although such waiver clauses are not legally enforceable, they may be practically may be effective in shielding the facility from lawsuit. Ambrogi points out that most contracts omit definitions of key terms such as the services covered by the daily rate; as a result, the monthly charge incurred often exceeds that explained as the basic daily rate.

Some agreements even contain clauses that conflict with the Bill of Rights. The most common clause requires residents to agree in advance to a broad range of medical treatment and diagnostic procedures (Ambrogi and Gerard 1986). These blanket consents allegedly empower the institution's staff to diagnose or treat conditions on the basis of their professional discretion without the need for any further decision by the elder. Also, some contracts are required to be signed by a so-called "responsible party" or "guarantor," who assumes not only personal financial liability of the elder as a requirement of admission, but medical decision-making authority; such a practice seems to violate statutory procedures regarding surrogate health care decisionmaking in many states and fundamentally abridges the right of elders to fully informed consent. A financial guarantor may, in fact, not even be the legal guardian of the patient, yet their signature on an admission agreement is taken to constitute blanket consent. Ambrogi reports that other rights are regularly infringed on in admission agreements: confidentiality of medical records and elders' right of access to them, the right to patronize a pharmacy of one's choice, the right to receive visitors of all ages at reasonable times, the right to privacy with respect to photographs, the right to reasonable policies regarding smoking and personal furnishings, and the right to access to nonfacility food and drink (1990: 74).

The language of rights is undeniably significant here. To have a right to x, however, does not mean that it is morally good to pursue x or to exercise x under any and all circumstances. It is important that the distinction between possessing a right and the morally justified exercising of a right not be overlooked. For example, though an elder has a right to refuse institutionalization in order to protect her sense of negative freedom, to do so in the face of family concern and her inability to care for herself in any minimally adequate sense requires justification *in addition to* appeal to the individual's right to do so. The right establishes what is *morally permitted*; it does not establish that its own exercise is *morally justified* in the circumstances. Insisting on basic rights in the admissions process and the protection of legal rights during institutionalization must not obscure the fact that the ethically defensible exercise of rights, whatever they may be, is itself a valid question, a point that indicates the inherent limitations associated with predicating an ethics of long-term care entirely on considerations of negative freedom.

The Use of Restraints

The presence of these admission practices nevertheless reinforces the lure of negative freedom and the values of self-determination and noninterference that are basic to our legal system and medical ethics. In a similar fashion, the use of physical restraints infringes on an obvious sense of autonomy as independence that liberals want to defend. Physical restraints are reported to be in wide use in nursing homes. These include restraining geri-chairs, waist, and "possey" restraints that tie the resident to a chair, as well as wrist restraints that are applied to residents at night and side rails that prevent residents from getting out of bed (Evans and Strumpf 1989). One argument frequently used to support the use of physical restraint involves the alleged institutional liability for injury. Some negligence cases are filed alleging the failure to prevent an institutionalized elder from falling or failure to use side rails (Kapp 1987). There is little evidence that institutions have been held liable for injury simply because they failed to employ physical restraint (Kapp 1985).

Andrew Jameton (1990) pointed out that there is a strong ethical presumption against using restraints. The presumption is not predicated on a very sophisticated understanding of freedom of action, but rather involves what he termed *elemental liberty*. In fact, the activities restricted by physical restraints are so basic that it is not easy to distinguish the ability to engage in the activities and the ability to make choices about engaging in them. The former is more a matter of physical competence and the latter mental competence, but with respect to activities like walking, sitting, standing, the two competencies merge. To be physically restrained is both to be rendered physically unable to act and so unable to make a meaningful choice regarding action (Jameton 1990: 167). On this view, then, there is a basic presumption against the use of restraints that derives from the most basic understanding of autonomy as negative freedom.

Restraints also increase a person's vulnerability to harm, exploitation, and neglect. They restrict physical motion and so the ability of an elder to protect oneself. In some instances, they constitute a danger to the elder. Perhaps more important, physical restraint is only one method among others that might be used to deal with a specific problem. Changing the structure of the environment (Cohen and Weisman 1990) can also obviate problems that are sometimes wrongly attributed to the elder. One might, for example, lower a bed as close to the floor as possible if the protective rails make the elder anxious (Blakeslee, Goldman, Papougenis 1990).

Jameton pointed out that a crucial element in the ethics of the use of restraints involves the degree of voluntariness involved. Seat belts provide a good contrast to restraints. Not only does their use serve life and health, it serves the choice of safety over risk. In the case of nursing home use of restraints, however, it is often difficult to sort out the level of voluntariness involved, in part, because of a background of involuntary admission, physical and mental impairments, and the profound control by staff of the rules and activities of daily life. For these reasons, appeal to the liberal principle of noninterference helps to establish the basic ethical presumption against using restraints in the first place. The complication is that presumptions can be overridden. Good reasons exist for using restraints in some circumstances. The initial appeal of negative freedom is thereby considerably diminished. The ethically interesting, and indeed perplexing, questions arise when we step beyond this basic presumption. Jameton (1990) argued that six factors are ethically relevant in making decisions to restrain elders: the frequency and intensity of danger posed to others, the frequency and intensity of danger posed to self, the wishes of the elder, the mental competence of the elder, the comfort of the elder with the restraints, and the wishes of the family. Considering these factors is clearly a step beyond the mere appeal to negative autonomy and toward more positive visions of what it means to be a moral agent with responsibilities to self and others, yet vulnerable as well. The usual outcome of the appeal to negative freedom is to stymie work toward achieving this positive account.

Simply prohibiting the use of restraints without further analysis and discussion is not ethically sufficient because restraints are a response to genuine problems in the care of some elders. The issues of assuring safety and preventing injury must be accounted for in any adequate response. One needs to question the meaning of wandering and the significance of falls in order to develop positive approaches to the management of these problems that are predicated on autonomy as a moral ideal. Be that as it may, what is most important is the way that an expansive liberal reading of autonomy can usurp other considerations when extended beyond its proper bounds.

The Perils of Liberal Theory

One significant deficiency with the standard liberal view of autonomy for long-term care is that it supports an abstract view of persons as independent, self-sufficient centers of decisionmaking. In a sense, such individuals become absolute centers of decisionmaking. Hence, practical dilemmas seem always to be handled inadequately because the absolute, abstract appeal of autonomy trumps other legitimate concerns. One consequence is that individuals express or are seen to express preferences and decisions that they take to be absolutely binding in all relationships (Toulmin 1981). No wonder, then, that disagreements often result in conflicts and disputes that cannot be settled by appeal to further principles, shared belief, or rational discourse and negotiation. Autonomy thus becomes more an obsession than a moral principle (Callahan 1984).

This cultural fixation on autonomy has profound implications on the way that medical ethics has developed featuring considerations of patient rights. The right to informed consent, for example, deriving from the liberal principle of autonomy constrains medical intervention unless explicit consent is given. In compromised and debilitated patients suffering from confusion, however, explicit consent is often not forthcoming. Anxiety about death or dependence on medical treatment sometimes prompts patients to refuse even highly beneficial and relatively risk-free interventions. As interpreted by critics of liberal theory, this is so because liberalism requires and defends such outcomes on ethical grounds. That interpretation is neither required nor justified.

Since the requirement of consent derives from the principle of autonomy, it is often treated as ethically unquestionable, though it is easy to see that this is wrong. Steven H. Miles described the case of his ninety-four-year-old great aunt who refused cataract surgery despite assurances that it was a minor, outpatient procedure (Miles 1988). Her refusal was related to her belief that if she went to the hospital she would die, as did her mother fifty years earlier from a septic gallbladder. Miles, a physician, felt torn between respecting his aunt's autonomy and her right to be free from the interference of strangers on the one hand and his sense of responsibility and desire to help as a nephew on the other. As Miles expressed it,

> as an absolute, autonomy reveals an impoverished view of how we live and are sustained in moral communities. On balance, the "autonomy ethic" serves many persons well. But, the epitaph of "It's their responsibility" is a facile way to blame those not served by this standard and excuse us from their need for our care. (1988: 2583)

Although this example is, strictly speaking, an instance of an acute care decision, it should not be forgotten that such crises are not altogether uncommon for elders in long-term care. In such situations the family members or guardians are asked to make decisions on behalf of the elder. Leaving aside the question of whether the patient is presently competent or not, one can ask, "Does autonomy afford any substantive moral guidance for such decisions?" On the model of autonomy as negative freedom, the answer is clearly not. Even when the patient is competent, as in Miles's case, autonomy affords a justification that is satisfactory more in the abstract than in a reality. In fact, what is at the heart of Miles's case is the morally destitute position marked by the sheer lack of fundamental concern or sympathy for the other that standard understandings of the meaning of autonomy seem to offer. If autonomy is to be a relevant consideration in such cases, a positive account will be necessary to augment the substantive basis for decisionmaking.

Analogous problems occur in the everyday world of long-term care (Kane and Caplan 1990). Although the consequences of honoring a putatively autonomous choice or providing care are less dramatic, they are nonetheless ethically significant. For example, how is autonomy relevant to deciding degrees and kinds of "protections," including restraints, for elders who are confused, cognitively impaired, or demented? Is it more important to afford institutionalized elders choices, for example, from a range of routine in-house social activities, such as bingo, crafts, or the once-a-month communal birthday party, or is it more important that the options available be meaningful for the particular elders involved? Playing bingo may be one of the few regular group activities available for nonambulatory elders; yet, if bingo (or other organized social activities) are seen by a particular elder as meaningless or even offensive, then the very act of affording the choice, including the opportunity to consider the option and freely deciding whether or not to attend, could diminish, even though subtly, the elder's sense of self-worth and magnify the alienation. Although such an outcome is regrettable, is it a problem of autonomy?

When an elder prefers to sit in a nearby park where casual encounters are routinely possible, but the nursing home does not afford access, especially for one who does not ambulate, then is the existence of a choice between bingo or other activities within the nursing home a response that adequately respects autonomy? If the elder in question suffers from confusional states, is a trip to the park, no matter how much the elder insists on it, a defensible option that should be honored just because it is the choice of the elder? Are there other factors to consider and appeal to besides the mere fact of choice or preference in respecting autonomy? Responses that simply insist on autonomy as the free exercise of choice in these examples to the exclusion of other factors seem quite unsatisfactory, though as yet it is not evident why this should be true; or, if it is true, what it has to do with autonomy.

Implied in the foregoing remarks is the view that if autonomy as negative freedom is not restricted to the political/legal realm, but is permitted to canonically define ethics, then the practical problems associated with long-term care will be oversimplified. The rich terrain of the everyday world of long-term care will be flattened and made more monotonous than it now appears. Even if we pursue the ideal of autonomy as negative freedom for elders through various procedural devices (such as nursing home preadmission agreements), the deeper ethical questions of the human meaning of autonomy and its apparent loss or alteration in old age are left to one side. Addressing these questions, however, seems an essential requirement of a treatment of autonomy that purports to adequately reflect the reality of long-term care.

The concept of negative freedom, like a herd of cattle when allowed to roam outside its normal range, inevitably tramples without discrimination both the flowers and weeds of everyday life. The widespread cultural belief that reference to independence and noninterference exhausts all that can be meaningfully said about autonomy simply cannot be accepted. Such a view, some would say, reflects the liberal idolatry of the individual, though such idolatry may be more the symptom than the cause. One intellectually serious reaction to this attitude and its under-lying cultural values has been the search for an alternative ethic, one that deci-sively rejects the liberal value of autonomy as independence. Much of this effort has been conducted under the emblem of communitarianism.

Communitarianism and the Contextualist Alternative

Communitarianism is a motley movement that broadly involves a critique of lib-eral individualism and autonomy, as well as the permissiveness that it promotes, and appeals to ideas and ideals of community, tradition, and virtue as foundational elements in ethics (Bellah *et al.* 1985; Hauerwas 1981; MacIntyre 1981; 1988; Perry 1988; Sandel 1982). Communitarians typically argue that autonomy is not a definitive value nor is it universally accepted; it is a product of a certain historical epoch, the Enlightenment or Age of Modernity. For this reason, among many, they claim that the alleged universal and nonsectarian quality attributed to autonomy by liberal theorists is largely a matter of historical amnesia. Communitarians typically argue for a view of ethics that focuses on the formation of character rather than the possession of rights and obligations. Ethics thus is understood primarily in terms of virtues that themselves are understood as related to a teleological unity of life that is anchored in the concept of a tradition. Individual selves are regarded as the subject of a history that is communal. The self is thus essentially bound up with membership in communities, such as those of family, neighborhood, city, and tribe or nation. That means that the self finds its moral identity in and through membership in these various communities. In a sense, then, individuals are never unformed, but exist primarily through identifications with others. For this to occur, communitarians frequently assume that a tradition requires a high degree of moral consensus not just about particular beliefs and values, but about the final pur-poses and nature of human life (MacIntyre 1988). Individuals fit within this all-encompassing structure as episodes in a story fit within a larger narrative struc-ture. Hence, individual human lives have unity insofar as they exhibit a kind of narrative structure.

Individuals are understood in terms of the kind of lives they live comparable with the kind of stories their lives tell about them. But the kind of stories that are open to individuals to exhibit in their lives is not infinite, according to com-munitarians; rather, there is a specific set of alternatives limited by a community's particular and determinate beliefs about the ultimate purpose of human life. These beliefs define the shared tradition that gives form and purpose to individual exist-ence. The final purpose and nature of human life is seen as essentially articulated in tradition which is the foundational repository of authority for making ultimate moral judgments. In other words, there is an implicit claim that tradition has a privileged and not a relative access to this transcendent truth.

An implication of communitarian thought is that individualism and autonomy are deficient ideals because they sever individuals from the very cultural and his-torical tradition that persons need to sustain themselves as moral agents. Communitarians often insist that instead of free choice and independence, acceptance of the authority of tradition or of communal authorities should be encouraged. Persons are said to realize their true nature and purpose only insofar as they exhibit character traits and virtues that allow participation in the wider reality of tradition and community. To be moral is to place oneself in the bosom of the larger community because only the community can provide the ultimate moral meaning of human life and action. An important implication of these views is that the transcendent reality of human nature is available as a source and guide for the ethical life of individuals only as authoritatively interpreted by the community (Hauerwas 1982; Veatch 1982).

Communitarianism exhibits one seriously deficient philosophical assumption that renders it a nonviable option, namely, its view that a contextual justification of moral beliefs or actions is completely incapable of securing their objectivity (Larmore 1987: 27–35). Communitarians regularly assume that the objectivity of a particular moral belief can be established only if the whole of our moral beliefs can be justified, only if we can show that *as a whole* they justify or make sense of human action by reference to an extramoral telos. This belief is, in effect, an epistemological foundationalism carried over to the realm of morality (Larmore 1987: 29). The requirement that any belief is justified only if the belief as a whole is justified is a tremendously difficult requirement for any theory to meet, including communitarianism. No wonder, then, that no communitarian account has really succeeded in establishing this objectivity. Given the diversity of knowledge and traditions to which communitarians themselves appeal, such an outcome is inevitable, though it is not adequately acknowledged by these thinkers.

The concept of tradition is appealed to, but tradition so regarded is an abstraction rather than a concrete, actual historical entity. The latter seldom is substantively systemic and rational *as a whole*. In fact, there are good reasons to doubt whether claims about tradition *simpliciter* have anything more than rhetorical or argumentative significance. In any event, according to communitarians, tradition is something within which one lives; it is not something that one puts on for the occasion like a suit of clothes. It is conveniently overlooked that real traditions frequently and essentially include dissent, so if dissent is to be forestalled for fear that it lead to anarchy, then appeal to tradition really amounts to an appeal to authority to settle matters of contemporary debate. Indeed, the authority appealed to is powerful enough to impose orthodoxy and foreclose discussion and debate.

Such a line of argument is logically defective because it displays a circularity of reasoning. It will not do simply to insist that a holistic vision or metaphysical view of the final ends or purposes of humanity is required because that is precisely what is in dispute between communitarians and liberals. Tradition regarded abstractly is used to bludgeon the liberal alternative while all-too-frequently it is overlooked that liberalism, too, can be regarded as a tradition (MacIntyre 1988).

The view that an authoritative foundation is necessary, and that such a foundation is ultimately metaphysical or substantive, seems a common prerequisite for communitarian accounts. Although this kind of commitment is shared with expresist brands of liberalism, the *modus vivendi*, contextualist, or pragmatic versions seem comfortable with the absence of such substantive anchors. That is not to say that these views endorse relativism, but they do acknowledge that the modern sense of foundation articulated in the work of Descartes is but one side of modern thought (Toulmin 1990). Indeed, the need felt for a foundation or anchor expresses a certain insecurity that is characteristic of modern thinking, though it is not at all clear why absolute foundations or first principles are needed to philosophically articulate a coherent world view.

One serious criticism of liberalism made by communitarians is that the liberal view of autonomy commits one to relativism or subjectivism such that objectivity of moral belief becomes impossible to secure. In the practical context, this amounts to the claim that the only ethics possible is therefore a situational ethics, implying an objectionable relativism. The only way to avoid such relativism, communitarians insist, is to adhere to the authority of tradition and community. Communitarianism typically rejects the view that ethics is truly a distinct realm; it rejects the idea that we attain our real humanity only in and through morality. Instead, communitarians often want to reestablish particular theological views, for example, the view that morality is the route to salvation. Hence, ethics is made dependent on religion. Such alternatives are properly rejected on liberal grounds as being at least potentially coercive or oppressive (Engelhardt 1991). Tyranny, not community, is often the result of such imposed religious visions of the good life, as history repeatedly demonstrates.

Both the liberal defense of the primacy of negative freedom in the sphere of ethics and the communitarian insistence on the primacy of tradition and community over individuals exhibit a common defect. Embracing tradition and community as *ultimate* sources of authority seems to commit the same kind of mistake attributed by communitarians to liberal thought, namely, of insisting on an absolute authority; the difference is that communitarians do so on the side of the community rather than the individual. Both of these extreme views need to be rejected. The alternative to both absolutistic liberal and communitarian thought is *contextualism*, namely, the view that actions and beliefs can be justified in a rationally defensible way without having to appeal to absolute principles or theories.

Contextualism is the view that morality is properly concerned with the life of human beings who exist as finite, social creatures engaged in particular existential settings and projects. This means that justification itself is seen as a human endeavor and one that is local. There is no absolute, privileged, or completely objective standpoint from which to settle ethical disputes once and for all. To be sure, such an absolute view of justification is implicit in much of the liberal tradition and is rightly targeted by communitarian critics. Justification in the eyes of these liberal thinkers inevitably involves a relativism of individuals not because there is no absolute basis for justification of belief, but because the basis lies with each independent individual. Communitarian critics themselves, perhaps more than is usually recognized, are heirs of liberal, post-Enlightenment thinking; they share an unbridled faith in certainty, though explicated in terms of community or tradition rather than the individual. The contextualist view is differentiated from both the liberal insistence on the primacy of negative freedom and its corollary of the individual as the final arbiter in moral matters as well as the communitarian belief in the final authority of tradition and community.

The view of contextualism is not new. Aristotle, too, had argued that there are no "essences" in the realm of ethics. There could, therefore, be no basis for any scientifically rigorous theory of ethics and no basis for any absolute principles of ethics. Practical reasoning in ethics, as in other practical contexts, such as clinical medicine, is essentially a matter of judgment. The exercise of judgment involves weighing and considering different alternatives. It is never simply a matter of formally deducing conclusions from strict or self-evident axioms or rules. At the basis of my reservations regarding both liberal theory and communitarian thought are serious reservations about the adequacy of the theory of ethics to which these views seem committed. This is admittedly no small matter, though it need not detain us at present since I return to this point after developing a positive view of autonomy.

Practical Implications of the Debate over the Foundation of Ethics

The debate over the nature of autonomy and its relation to morality is not only theoretically interesting and important, but also has practical implications for long-term care. As argued above, the liberal view of autonomy and its corollary articulation in legal rights is compatible with the criticism of that view when liberal theory is extended beyond its proper political bounds. It is thus possible to retain the positive features of the liberal view of autonomy and the legal protections afforded elderly individuals, while still criticizing these views for usurping the proper concerns of ethics in long-term care. One does not need to accept communitarian thought uncritically, particularly insofar as it tends to underestimate the significance of the liberal value of protecting the rights of individuals in the public or political/legal sphere and is committed to a sometimes naive foundationalism. Instead, one can look to an account of autonomy that captures some of the central tendencies and insights of communitarian thought, namely, that humans are social creatures who must be understood in terms of their concrete relations with one another and that tradition and community are important, though not absolute, sources of moral insight and guidance, without trying to secure a monistic or absolutistic vision of the good life.

The practical implication of this point is that the fabric of rights secured by the liberal concept of autonomy is left intact, though its application is made a matter of moral judgment and discretion. In the context of long-term care, the function of autonomy that remains vital is to provide procedural protections to assure that a range of alternative expressions of the best way to grow old, to handle disability, or to live out the last days of one's life are possible. This pluralistic outcome does not imply, as communitarians often (though wrongly) insist, that the foundations necessary for ethics or the moral life are eliminated. An absolutistic, foundationalist ethics is, to be sure, eliminated, but a contextual ethics, the only kind ultimately possible for finite beings, is retained. This may not satisfy most communitarians, but it can accommodate the central substantive contributions of communitarian thought to contemporary ethics. The crucial insight on which proponents of communitarianism properly insist is unequivocally retained, namely, that the moral life

is essentially social and that persons are not atomistic, self-centered, rational decision makers, but selves formed by a living tradition and culture. Moral agents by
definition exhibit more than freedom of action or choice; they manifest character
and virtues. Communitarians are correct because the expansive version of autonomy
as negative freedom is self-defeating generally and certainly unhelpful and unwork-
able in the context of long-term care. Fortunately, nothing in liberal theory, properly interpreted, logically requires such an extreme conclusion anyway. So unless
one wishes to joust with straw men, it seems frivolous to tarry any longer on these
points.

The proper interpretation of the liberal theory of autonomy is a contextualist
defense of liberalism that restricts the individualistic view of negative freedom to
the political/legal realm. Positive concepts of autonomy are not only possible but
necessary for ethics. Communitarian thought contributes much to the contemporary
establishment of ethics. An account of the nature of the moral life that is compatible with a restricted liberal theory is thus possible; such an account is also compatible with the broad outlines of communitarian views regarding the nature of persons
as historical and social beings and the importance of character and virtue in ethics.
These contributions are important because they help prevent turning ethics into the
play of principles that have the sole purpose of regulating interactions among strangers
(Toulmin 1981). The incursion of such an "ethic of strangers" into health care has
had the effect of reinterpreting caring, intimacy, and other emotional attachments
as prima facie evidence of objectionably paternalistic behavior. It would be most
unfortunate if an ethics of long-term care were to repeat these mistakes.

Respect for autonomy as independence is important in those settings in which
the language of rights and principles of equity and equality are properly central.
Accepting this point, however, does not make the liberal principle of autonomy
and the language of rights the primary concepts of ethics in other situations that
involve intimacy or concrete and genuine moral conflict, complexity, and tragedy. If the primary function of the principle of autonomy was to make sense of
and justify an adversarial legal system that addresses conflictual interactions
between strangers, what would happen in situations in which the psychological
outcomes were the most damaging and serious, such as in situations of conflict
involving the care of children or elders? Stephen Toulmin (1981) pointed out that
in just such areas as family law, other nations (e.g., West Germany) have chosen
to handle disputes through arbitration rather than through litigation, in chambers
rather than in open court, to provide as much room as possible for discretion. The
focus on arbitration rather than litigation and on judgmental discretion rather than
rigorism in the application of principles is especially significant because it rightly
indicates that the ethics of relationships with intimates, such as family members
or acquaintances, is fundamentally different from moral relationships with complete strangers. If so, important implications follow for the ethics of long-term care
in which intimacy is an important feature.

Long-term care is not adequately understood if it is restricted to the ethics
of relationships between strangers. Certainly such relations exist and are probably
unavoidable in some long-term care situations. In most long-term care, however,
when strangers enter these relationships, degrees of intimacy and familiarity develop

as the inevitable outcomes of continuous interaction. Indeed, when they fail to develop, something is basically amiss in the social environment of caregiving. Hence, it is critically important to assess what "respect for autonomy" can mean in circumstances that deviate significantly from the model assumed by the dominant view of autonomy as negative freedom or independence.

One way to develop these points preliminarily is to consider how the view of autonomy as independence (and the view of inviolate patient rights that derives therefrom) is related to assumptions about the nature of medicine and health care. I return to this analysis in Chapter 3, but an anticipatory discussion is not inappropriate at this point. Simply put, it appears that autonomy conceived in terms of independence is recommended by certain acute care situations that paradigmatically support the extension of the political/legal view of autonomy into medical ethics. In much of medical ethics, the standard or paradigm cases and problems seem to be oriented to dramatic conflictual so-called four-alarm cases (McCullough and Wear 1985: 296–97). Conflict and disagreement are predominate and patients (as well as families) seem to become pawns in the hands of a powerful and impersonal system of medical care. It is at least arguable that long-term care requires a different paradigm or framework (Agich 1990c) because such dramatic cases of conflict are less evident in long-term care or because exclusive attention to such cases diverts attention from more pervasive, interstitial aspects of everyday life that should be the focus of attention (Kane and Caplan 1990). Indeed, one by-product of a serious examination of the ethics of long-term care might be the development of a different orientation toward medical ethics generally, one that leads away from a fixation on autonomy as independence. One point, however, is clear: if the issue is the mundane aspects of long-term care, then rights language does not provide a very apt tool for shaping these concerns.

Conflict and Conversation

Preliminary to developing an alternative framework for assessing autonomy in long-term care, it is important to appreciate how certain commitments of the liberal view of autonomy that I have defended also support the view that individuals are best understood in social terms, rather than as atomistic, rational decision makers. It is important to make clear that the liberal view is badly represented by the libertarian, individualistic extreme; the liberal view of autonomy properly interpreted can without inconsistency regard individuals as historical, social beings consistent with the central focus of communitarian thought. One way to establish this point is to consider the logical requirements of neutrality and toleration. As Larmore put it,

> neutrality is simply a means of accommodation. It is a stance that we adopt in order to solve a specific problem to which our various commitments give rise, and so it is not a stance that expresses our full understanding of our purposes. It establishes a modus vivendi between persons whose ultimate ideals do not coincide. (1987: 74)

Several considerations recommend such a stance.

First, the norm of rational conversation requires that if we want to solve a problem but encounter disagreement about how to do so, we should retreat to neutral ground. Second, besides a desire for civil peace and sympathy for those whose ideals are similar to ours, the norm of equal respect demands that we explain our proposals to those whom they will affect, even if we believe that they will disagree. Third, our own pursuit of some substantial ideal of the good life, it seems reasonable to believe, will be protected if others, with different ideals, also agree that common political principles must be sought from neutral ground. Importantly, none of these reasons calls for any weakening of our allegiance to our own beliefs and values or our own vision of the good life.

When confronted by irresolvable disagreement, individuals who wish to continue a discussion or conversation must retreat to a neutral ground with the hope of either resolving the dispute or bypassing it. This retreat to a neutral ground allows one to remain as convinced of the truth of one's views as before, but for the purposes of carrying on the conversation, one sets aside the absolute claim of these beliefs. In other words, the ideal or goal of "keeping the conversation going," which is motivated by the desire to achieve some reasoned agreement about how to solve the problem at hand, gives substantive force to the ideal of neutrality (Larmore 1987: 53). For this to occur, at least two criteria must be met: first, the conditions necessary for conversation, namely, the prerequisites for communicative interaction, must be available, and, second, the desire or commitment to solve the problem at hand through reasoned agreement must override the tendency to use force to end the impasse. These conditions posit a view of individuals as historical, social beings who must, by their very nature, live together and interact.

Reason, rather than force, is compelling not because it is more effective, all things considered, but because it preserves the very conditions of interaction, whereas force destroys the social fabric necessary for human beings to be truly human. Although one may "win" a dispute by force, for example, by killing one's opponent, such a maneuver makes impossible the conditions that sustain human beings in historical and social relationships. One need only consider the problems, for example, in Lebanon, Israel's occupied territories, or Yugoslavia to see the difficulty that reliance on force engenders. Similarly, one need only look to the sorry state of many long-term care settings that rely on staff authority and power to "manage" their charges for ready examples of the practical consequences of this view. It is worth noting that typically reliance on coercion and force does not so much make human social existence impossible as reduce the qualitative possibilities, a consequence that should nonetheless be regarded as of equal ethical importance.

The Function of Rights

Appeals to autonomy often are made in situations of conflict in long-term care, such as over decisions to institutionalize, to increase levels of skilled care, or to begin, withhold, or withdraw life-prolonging medical technologies. Such appeals undoubtedly serve the important function in these contexts of curbing the pretensions and power of health care providers. Prominent in this process of appeal is the language of rights: for example, the right to refuse treatment, the right to informed consent, the right of self-determination. The language of rights has several features that concretely illustrate the general features of the liberal concept of autonomy, especially as it is employed in medical ethics. To be sure, rights do offer protection to individuals from the impersonal decisionmaking of health care institutions and health professionals who hold a disproportionate share of power. A claim to rights thus is often a strong moral counterweight to a line of decision-making that rests on, for example, what the rules of an institution require, what is customary in the profession or institution, or what the practitioner usually does in such cases (Agich 1982). This feature is undoubtedly important, but it comes into play and is significant primarily when controversy ensues or conflict arises. The language of rights does not tell how to avoid these circumstances, nor does it seem able to satisfactorily settle true cases of ethical conflict or dilemma.

Examples of true ethical dilemmas involve fundamental conflicts of principle or value. Such cases are not settled simply by insisting on one principle over and against its competition, yet the language of rights gives the impression that if one simply honors a valid right, then the tragedy of having to make a moral judgment is avoided because ethics simply, at rock bottom, requires that the right be upheld. This implication is supported by three important logical properties that characterize rights.

First, rights claims are unique moral claims in that they are peremptory: they are absolute and bar further debate or discussion; they cannot be changed, delayed, or denied. When a person's rights are involved, many sorts of action are authorized that would otherwise be impermissible (Ladd 1978: 16). For example, it is wrong to harm another person, yet if Mr. Jones tries to take my wallet, I am justified in physically preventing him from doing so even if my actions cause him harm. Even though it is morally wrong to kill, my own right to life justifies my efforts to defend myself even to the extent of causing my assailant mortal harm. Second, because rights are appealed to when the person against whom the right is asserted threatens, neglects, or otherwise appears unwilling to accede to one's requests, needs, or demands, they assume that an adversarial relationship exists between the parties involved (Ladd 1978: 17; Wellman 1985: 102). Third, it is important to note that an individual possesses a right if he can choose not to exercise it. In this sense, rights are a reflection of the concept of a person as free and capable of making decisions. Decision-making competence or capacity is simply presumed. More important for present purposes, it is also presumed that the choices available to the rights possessor are in some broad sense desirable or even sensible. The right is simply assumed to enable a choice that ranges over alternative courses of action that are assumed to be broadly "acceptable." That, of course, need not be the case. It is a theoretical fiction that the choices afforded by a right are unproblematic just so long as they are afforded by a valid right, whereas in fact everyday experience is rife with examples in which this does not seem to be the case. A simple example can illustrate this point.

I have a meal ticket to a cafeteria that affords an extensive menu for lunch. One day each of the main courses, desserts, and soups contains milk or milk products to which I am allergic. My right to choose from among the offerings is unfettered, but my actual choice is burdened with the consequences of a known food allergy; alternatively, my choice might be constrained by religion-based dietary restrictions or simply by my preferences. In either of these situations, I have a right to choose guaranteed by my legitimate possession of a meal ticket even though each of the choices available is problematic for me. Rights advocates might be quick to point out, however, that this is not much of an objection since I retain other rights that give me other options, including the liberty right to forego using my meal ticket. This is undoubtedly true, but the important point is that the attention to rights tends to adjust the focus of analysis in such a way that the existential or actual detail is lost, namely, that the cafeteria's offerings are inadequate or insensitive to the dietary needs of at least one of its patrons. Were the management of the cafeteria simply to insist that my freedom to eat in the establishment is unaltered by the day's offerings seems to miss the point at issue, namely, that at least one patron is unable to partake of what may be well-prepared and wholesome food. Pointing this out involves no necessary criticism of the cafeteria nor does it carry any implication that is helpfully expressed in terms of my right to eat in the establishment. The example points, instead, to the fact that the language of rights is largely irrelevant to what is problematic in the actual circumstances, that is, my inability to eat in the cafeteria despite my possession of a meal ticket. Instead of being a matter of honoring or enforcing a set of rights claims, the case points to other dimensions that are penumbral on the rights-dominated approach. In certain cases, these dimensions are revealed through the application of other ethical concepts, such as responsibility (Agich 1982). In all of these concrete examples, the exercise of practical judgment is indispensable.

Rights are typically seen as important because of their tie to autonomy understood in terms of nonintervention or noninterference. That is, rights are designed to afford individuals protection from the intrusion of others. The assumption seems to be that individuals need such protection because individuals as persons are best understood on their own or in their own terms, and that ethics is best understood as the effort to protect the freedom of choice. In effect, persons are construed as social and moral atoms in that they are represented without significant reference to their own developmental history, personal values, or relationships with others. Human relationships are thereby taken to be a secondary aspect of being a person for purposes of the theory. Relationships are considered only insofar as they problematically represent intrusion on the solitude of individuals, a condition that is taken to be both normal and normative. The truly autonomous individual is assumed to exist in a steady state, in a state of rationality or competence. The psychological nature of competence or the complexity associated with spelling out the various ends or purposes that competence instrumentally serves is frequently forgotten or simply set to one side. In point of fact, the empirical concreteness of the individual is nowhere to be found. Instead, the view becomes, as Thomas Nagel (1986) so-aptly expressed it, "the view from nowhere."

Finally, the emphasis on rights focuses attention on actions such as the delivery of goods and services that are either strictly forbidden or required. The domain of ethics is thus constricted; actions that are ethically permissible, including much of the domain of virtue, are viewed as having only peripheral relevance. Because they are not proscribed nor required as a matter of right, such actions are of little interest. Yet if the central concern guiding long-term care involves caring for frail and dependent elders, it would seem that the focus should be on what is ethically optimal, not simply on what is proscribed. Many things are ethically good that are not obligatory as a matter of someone's possession of a valid right. A child may not have a right to the love and care of his parents, yet the bestowal of love and care is surely required of parents nonetheless.

Limitations of Rights

In Kantian terms, rights involve "perfect" duties, duties that are strict and deter-minate: perfect duties justify enforcement, that is, morally justify forcing others to honor the right possessed. This means that moral judgment, the concrete weighing of circumstances and considering the actual concrete existential situation, is hardly encouraged. Instead, morality is conceived to consist in simply honoring valid rights claims no matter whether doing so conflicts with other moral goods or other val-ues. Other actions such as caring, compassion, or solicitude are relegated to a less significant or, indeed, a peripheral status. In general, what Kant termed *imperfect duties*, that is, duties that we all have as moral agents, such as the duty to be chari-table or to be compassionate, are ignored. They are ignored precisely because they cannot be enforced as a matter of rights. One cannot force someone to be compas-sionate. Instead, one must educate or develop the character traits essential for the kind of caregiving that one wants to see in relationships such as parent-child or doctor-patient. Similarly, though charity is a general (imperfect) duty, it is inde-terminate. Each of us is obliged to be charitable, but the obligation of charity does not carry with it any specification of the precise actions or circumstances that satisfy it. There is a range of discretion for judgment in the choice of actions and circum-stances. To be sure, each of us reveal character traits and ideals in our choices, and these may be matters for ethical analysis and discussion, but our charitable actions are not corollaries of anyone's entitlement. Naturally, if situations of con-flict comprise the paradigm, then concern for character will no doubt appear pal-lid in contrast to the robust legalistic rectitude afforded by rights language.

On the basis of the assumption associated with rights, individuals are repre-sented in contractual (based on explicit agreement) or quasi-contractual (based on assumed or implicit agreement) terms and human relationships are generally defined in static and impersonal terms. As a result, respect for persons means respecting individuals abstractly as autonomous, independent, mature (competent), and static centers of decisionmaking and choice. Persons are "respected" from an emotional distance; real, actual individuals with life histories and personal stories are simply nowhere to be found! An implication of this view is that one main task of ethics comes to involve ordering, weighing, or reconciling different values or interests. Hence, it should not surprise anyone to recognize that ethics has adopted avail-able models for conducting such ordering and weighing from economics. The utili-tarian calculus and contemporary applications of decision analysis have their roots in economic thinking. Indeed, the original sense of the term *value* and its cognate *worth* was monetary value. Only subsequently did the word take on the sense of the "goodness of something." In the modern world, metaphors drawn from economics dominate our thinking about questions of value and the good so much that we may have difficulty in appreciating the respects in which ethical value has formal properties that are different from monetary value (Whitbeck 1985: 184–85).

It is easy to recognize the implications of this association. Within the framework of the liberal concept of autonomy, it is assumed that values can be ordered and sometimes quantified and maximized. The process of decisionmaking is thought to be eminently rational. Choice consists in the weighing of values and preferences that individuals have. Whether the values and preferences are worth having in the sense of "morally good" or "morally appropriate or proper" independent of the quantitatively inspired sense of monetary value is an issue that makes little sense in this setting. Accordingly, ethics becomes involved with the task of discovering the rules that maximize the good or finding the fairest tradeoff among competing values. As a result, appeals to autonomy usually take two forms. Those who are autonomous are allowed to make health care decisions on their own behalf free of any coercion or limitations because their right to do so "trumps" all other considerations (Dworkin 1977), and those who do not possess the quality of autonomy (such as severely dependent, sick, and debilitated persons) may have decisions made on their behalf by surrogate decision makers.

It is interesting, and perhaps ironic, that surrogate decisionmaking has assumed such importance in health care decisions, but it is not surprising given the influence of legalistic thinking in medical ethics (Buchanan and Brock 1989). On the liberal model of autonomy, individuals must possess minimal communication skills, minimal evidence of rationality, and minimum ability to comprehend the realities of their personal and social situation. Unfortunately, these requirements are often not met in medicine, particularly not in individuals requiring institutional long-term care. Since autonomy is the central and dominant concept that defines what medical ethics is, the alternatives are limited. A myth or fiction of decisionmaking (hypothetically) by the patient is created to fill the void. Surrogate decisionmaking thus carries the concept of autonomy as negative freedom to its logical conclusion: if individuals are, as autonomy seems to require, centers of impersonal, rational decisionmaking, then such decisionmaking can, indeed must, be exercised by others when the individuals cannot do so themselves. The only compelling question is really a procedural question, namely, who has the authority to exercise decisionmaking for another? Because of our deep suspicion of physicians and other health care providers, the consensus response is anyone closely situated to the patient, so long as it is not the physician or health care provider. Some rightly have found the logic of surrogate decisionmaking problematic (Buchanan 1983). At the very least, it is paradoxical and the paradox points to a systemic problem associated with the traditional view of autonomy as negative freedom, namely, that it assumes a rather abstract view of human persons. Before engaging that point, it will be useful to discuss a concern that is almost synonymous with the treatment of autonomy, that is, the problem of paternalism.

Paternalism and the Development of Persons

Although *paternalism* is a highly problematic term conveying extremely pejorative connotations, it has roots in a positive and essential feature of human development, namely, the parental nurturance of infants and children. Typical treatments of paternalism have not taken this connection seriously (exceptions include Douglas 1983; O'Neill 1984; Whitbeck 1985). In part, this is so because discussions of paternalism have been so strikingly influenced by what I have termed the liberal concept of autonomy. Another factor, however, complicates the discussion of paternalism in health care. Frequently, actions that are best described as beneficent, namely, actions undertaken without coercion to benefit a patient, are tarred with the brush of paternalism on the assumption that any action taken by a health professional must in some objectionable way involve the imposition of professional power (Whitbeck 1985: 181; Thomasma 1984: 911–12). This is both understandable and lamentable.

So-called agency ethics or professional medical ethics defines the primary obligation of the physician—and by extension all health care providers—as doing everything possible to enhance the patient's welfare (American College of Physicians 1984b: 266; Beauchamp and Childress 1983: 213; Daniels 1986: 1382; Fried 1978: 234; Judicial Council of the American Medical Association 1984: 3; Levinsky 1984: 1573; Pellegrino and Thomasma 1981: 275; Veatch 1981: 287). Indeed, some argue that concern for the patient's well-being or concern for justice is a more plausible foundation for medical ethics than autonomy (Childress 1990; Pellegrino and Thomasma 1988). Of course, it is not the only fundamental principle, as even defenders of professional medical ethics point out; the obligation to heal or benefit the patient acquires "a normative force only when health and healing are ranked as primary by both physician and patients" (Pellegrino and Thomasma 1981: 187). Nevertheless, the appeal to agency ethics and the professional obligation of beneficence is frequently advanced in the service of political ends—for example, in the debate over the introduction of procompetition and prospective payment into medicine. This line of argument misunderstands both the meaning and scope of a professional obligation of beneficence and the relationship between incentives and obligations (Agich 1986; 1987; 1990a; 1990b). In light of these confusions and the rhetorical ends to which appeal to the obligation of beneficence has been put, it is understandable that others have insisted that respect for persons and autonomy constitutes the only defensible secular and nonsectarian foundation for medical ethics (Engelhardt 1986). The prominence given the obligation of beneficence, of course, does not alone explain the counter appeal of autonomy, but it is true that the profoundest arguments in defense of patient autonomy and rights are squarely placed in the context of an analysis of power and authority. The fact that such debates are on-going clearly shows that the aim of subordinating autonomy to beneficence remains controversial.

In spite of the overriding regard for self-determination promoted by the concept of autonomy just discussed, it has been recognized that there are possible moral justifications for departing from strict adherence to the rule of noninterference. As mentioned above, the inability of individuals to exhibit even minimal evidence of decision-making capacity makes the demand to respect autonomy—which means respecting an independent decision-making capacity—moot. In addition, the recognition of the basic facts of human development provides a ready, if only inadequately appreciated, basis for overriding autonomy. The fact is that human beings are not all-at-once persons, but develop historically as biopsychosocial entities under the care of human parents. This care, necessary for human growth and development, importantly includes interventions and actions that seem to constrain the infant's desires, actions, or otherwise interfere with self-determination. This fact is evident even to the staunchest individualist. Parental care not only is necessary for the development of human persons, but also provides a basis for morally justifying actions that limit or hinder the self-determination of another for that person's own good. Such acts have been broadly labeled *paternalistic.*

Caroline Whitbeck (1985: 183) noted that most treatments of paternalism overlook this significant reference to human development and the dynamics of the relationship in which it occurs. In fact, most treatments are modeled on the role of the monarch in governing subjects, a role that is directed not toward making subjects into future monarchs but toward ensuring their survival and prosperity as subjects. She noted that this model can be traced at least to Aristotle and that it remarkably fails to include many of the central features of the parenting role. The focus instead is on the political relation of monarch to subject; no wonder, then, that the main concern is that of noninterference.

It is unfortunate that the sexist term *paternalism* has taken on such negative associations. Given the development of treatments of the parent-child relationship modeled on that of the monarch-subject from Aristotle onward, it is easy to see how public interactions shape the model that evolved. Unfortunately, the parent-child relationship is a relationship of intimacy in which paternal authority itself is a positive role that is certainly complemented by the nurturing, "maternal" role, but is in no way fundamentally opposed to it. If we have learned anything from empirical studies of child-rearing practices, it is that these essential functions can be enacted in various ways. Some involve delineation along typical (for Western thought and experience) sex-determined parenting roles, but there is no logical requirement that such be the case. Recent experience of American families with two working parents has led to a variety of seemingly novel adaptations. It is not uncommon in professional couples, for instance, for the sex-delineated maternal and paternal roles to undergo dynamic adjustment as careers unfold and the child matures. Furthermore, common sense tells us parental authority and nurturance are necessarily exercised by parents of either sex in the actual dynamic relations that constitute childrearing. Philosophers should be especially skeptical of stereotyped and static models. We must be careful not to speak of paternal authority and maternal nurturance as if they were sex-determined, mutually exclusive functions.

The concept of paternalism derives from the Latin *pater* because the fatherly role typically consists in protecting the children from harm and danger; the father does for the children what they cannot do for themselves, including interfering to restrict expressions of freedom that pose danger or risk of harm. The maternal role, on the other hand, is usually seen as nurturing. The mother nurtures the child from a state of total dependence to a state of increasing independence and responsibility. It is an active calling forth of the child, a positive role of facilitating development of the child's autonomy. The father figure is associated with authority; the mother, with affection. The former is a restraining influence; the latter, a liberating influence. Both, however, are essential components of parenting.

The question of the priority of the maternal or paternal role has surfaced in controversy over models of moral reasoning (Kittay and Meyers 1987). Lawrence Kohlberg (1971) proposed three levels of moral reasoning, each composed of two stages, moving from premoral to mature moral reasoning. Mature moral reasoning is illustrated by deontological reasoning, namely, the appeal to universal moral principles or roles that govern human action by respecting another person's rights. Carol Gilligan (1982; 1987), however, criticized Kohlberg's research because it is based exclusively on the experience of males. Her own research on female subjects yields a different model of responsibility or relationship that is not predicated on individual rights. Both models, however, seem prone to misuse. Kohlberg's categories, for example, were claimed to be applicable to all individuals (Rest *et al.* 1974) and Gilligan's work has been interpreted as arguing for the superiority of the female model (Saxton 1981), though there seems good reason to view each model as complementary to the other (Mahowald 1987: 24). Failure to appreciate the complementary, yet dynamic, interrelationship between these models yields a remarkably one-sided view of ethics.

The term *parentalism* has been proposed by some as a nonsexist substitute for the term *paternalism* (Benjamin and Curtis 1981: 48–58). Others have objected that the substitution of the neutral term of parenting fails to overcome the sexist implications of paternal and maternal roles and ignores the real contributions of women as women that are irreplaceable by men. Mary B. Mahowald, however, argued that these concerns are valid only as a critique of a narrow notion of parenting and family relationships that prevail in today's society. The narrow notion views parenting as either maternally or paternally accomplished by individuals, as taking place merely during the period in which children are chronically young, and as occurring in a relationship that is biologically parental or legally adoptive (1987: 28–29). Real parenting, and so parentalism, is in fact practiced by people who are not biological parents and, in some instances, is not practiced by those who are. Parenting thus is a behavior and attitude that involves nurturance and protection across the entire life span and that promotes autonomy of the other even beyond the point where the nurturer's interventions are needed or desirable (Mahowald 1987: 29). Because parenting involves both life-begetting and life-sustaining functions, as well as an understanding of life as an unfolding and developing process whose goal is the fulfillment of each individual's unique potential, parentalism is an apt ethical model for all human relationships. The middle-aged woman, for example, who cares for her elderly senile father assumes the role of parent, in this sense, by providing for his fundamental needs (the paternal role of protection) while encouraging as much autonomy as he is able to handle (the maternal role of nurturance).

When a balance is struck between the roles of nurturance and protection, the ideal parenting is achieved. For this reason, the term *parentalism* should be reserved for this essential unitary requirement of human development. Rather than making parentalism a nonsexist term for paternalism, the positive meanings associated with human growth and development should be preserved. Substituting the positive term *parentalism* for the pejorative term *paternalism* betrays a singular insensitivity to the significance of parenting in human development and a striking testimony to the uncritical acceptance of liberal rhetoric. As Thomas Halper observed:

> "Paternalism" typically is greeted with all the enthusiasm reserved for a dead mouse in a dustpan. So powerful, in fact, are the word's pejorative connotations that in common speech it performs double duty: it describes a phenomenon and signals our distaste for it, both at the same time. But this apparent economy is very costly, and the price is paid in terms of the vagueness, ambiguity, unexamined assumptions, and confusion. (1978: 331)

It seems evident to a degree that makes argument unnecessary that the actual situation of a person's life is seldom one of total dependence or total independence, but is a combination of these or interdependence. We are thus always candidates for both protective and nurturing influences: we have needs that require attention and capabilities to be respected and fostered. Moreover, the sequence of development is such that we may sometimes, even as adults, be more dependent than independent in our interdependence. As R. M. Hare (1972: 72–78) pointed out, the tension between protecting and nurturing is a false dichotomy or dilemma because the dynamic relation between decisions and principles that are involved in actual moral life precludes any elevation of protection or nurturance above the other. Hare drew a rather interesting and important conclusion from this observation:

> Many of the dark places of ethics become clear when we consider this dilemma in which parents are liable to find themselves. We have already noticed that, although principles have in the end to rest upon decisions of principle, decisions as such cannot be taught; only principles can be taught. It is the powerlessness of the parent to make for his son those many decisions of principle which the son during his future career will make, that gives moral language its characteristic shape. The only instrument which the parent possesses is moral education—the teaching of principles by example and precept, backed up by chastisement and other more up-to-date psychological methods. (1972: 75)

Hare also discussed the further dilemma that arises when moral education is primarily in terms of a fundamental choice between teaching principles or actual decisionmaking. He argued that the dilemma posed by these two extreme alternatives is plainly false. Clearly, said Hare, you must provide children with a solid basis of principles at the same time that you afford ample opportunity for making decisions on which those principles are based and by which they are modified, improved, adapted to changed circumstances, or even abandoned if they are found to be unsuited to new situations (1972: 76). There is no dichotomy between principles and decisions, but rather a dynamic relationship that is vastly misunderstood if we concentrate on one or the other.

The parent-child situation nonetheless does seem to provide one significant model for justifying departures from the rule of noninterference; yet, as Whitbeck argued, the developmental context and the dynamic character of the relationship governing parent-child interactions was necessarily excluded from consideration by the very assumptions underlying the liberal concept of autonomy (1985: 184). To rehabilitate the concept of autonomy as a guiding principle for long-term care thus requires an exploration of how persons actually develop and how ethical theory can accommodate actual autonomy in a positive vision.

From Paternalism to Parentalism

David Thomasma argued that acting in the "best interests" of another person means acting with respect for the other's personal independence and judgment (Thomasma 1984: 911). In so doing, autonomy is not *waived*. Illness and incapacity themselves impede freedom, so acting in another's best interests when they are ill need not be paternalistic. In cases in which the patient's competence is severely compromised, a common mistake, Thomasma insisted, is to identify or confuse beneficence with paternalism (1984: 911-12). Some go so far as to assert that "in theory the benefit principle assumes the waiving of autonomy" (Gadow 1980: 680), though no compelling argument has shown that this is the case. The tendency to shift from a consideration of beneficence (namely, acting to benefit the other or pursue the other's well-being) to a consideration of paternalism (namely, the imposition of a view of what constitutes the good for another *against* that other's own wishes) is a common enough mistake. In the case of dependent elders, Thomasma argued, illness and disability have already effaced the ability of the elder to choose for herself; hence, the appropriate criterion is that "the greater the dependence of the patient on others, the greater is the care that must be taken to act to enhance her well-being" (1984: 911). An analogous point is captured in the distinction between direct and delegated autonomy (Collopy 1988). *Direct autonomy* involves explicit decision and action as individual, independent agents; *delegated autonomy* involves the acceptance or authorization of the actions and decisions of others. Delegated autonomy can surely be seen as a loss of independence, and hence autonomy as negative freedom, but for frail elders the other option is to bear the full weight of unsupported independence. Delegated autonomy directs attention to the ethical character of long-term care, including its reciprocal nature, its characteristic response to vulnerability, and the dynamic interplay between competence and incompetence and control and freedom (Collopy 1988: 12; May 1982).

Often what is taken to be a problem of paternalism is really a problem of a failure of communication on the part of the health professional. As Whitbeck observed, physicians are often "guilty" not of paternalistic behavior toward patients but of beneficence toward patients (Whitbeck 1985: 181). Behavior can properly be described as paternalistic only if it results from a decision to override the autonomous choice of patients, but physicians usually do not make such judgments; instead, they often simply fail to communicate effectively with patients on matters with which they have difficulty dealing, such as death or medical uncertainty. This is compatible with the fact that medicine and, by extension, health care has historically been quite paternalistic (Buchanan 1981: 14; Childress 1982: 40; Veatch

1981: 15–26, 141–76). If these points are correct, then what becomes of the putative problem of paternalism in medicine generally and long-term care in particular?

In answering this question it is helpful to recall that freedom from interference remains an important value when confined to the political/legal sphere. Appeal to this sphere should be open whenever health care providers—or others who hold power over individuals—fail to exercise their power and authority responsibly. When that failure occurs is obviously a matter of some dispute. The claim that the more pervasive concern is beneficence not paternalism can be interpreted as a challenge to reinterpret the responsibilities implied by the care-giving role in a way that does not license care-givers to override patient rights.

In discussions of these matters, it is frequently assumed that the caregiver is a professional and that the relationship between caregiver and patient is a professional relationship. Professionals hold a special place in society. They have special privileges and authority from which derive specific powers over individuals. Whenever individuals are involved in relationships with health professionals, it is important to be clear whether the relationship is legalistically professional (that is, defined in terms of norms that regulate interactions between individuals with whom one does not share a basic viewpoint) or is another kind of human relationship that develops spontaneously on the basis of implicit and explicit promises, understandings, and fairly complex communicative interactions. If the latter circumstance comprises the caregiving, then even professional relationships will be amenable to analysis in terms that require a more concrete theory of autonomy.

The attitude that Thomasma described is clearly not strictly paternalism. It might better be described as *parentalism*, that is, the situation in which an affectively concerned caregiver strives to enhance the well-being, *including the autonomy*, of another dependent individual. In effect, parentalism could be the model for what has been called "autonomy respecting paternalism" (VanDeVeer 1986). Parentalism assumes that the dependence is not caused by the caregiver and that it is not sustained by the caregiver through any form of coercion, no matter how benevolently motivated. It also assumes that well-being is not imposed over the objection or free and competent choice of the dependent other. Parentalism has its roots in a phenomenon essential to being a human person, namely, that human persons do not spring into being fully formed as independent agents, but develop through psychosocial relations with human parents. It signals the essential interconnectedness of all human persons and points to the positive obligations that arise in such relationships. Parentalism also points to the fact that adult human beings are necessarily interdependent and that despite their maturity require nurturance. They exist as persons through actions in the common and shared world of everyday life. The problem of autonomy is badly articulated if it is simply juxtaposed to paternalism because paternalism classically involves a thin view of persons as independent agents. Mill's important reflections *On Liberty* (1978) are developed under the simplifying assumption that the agent is in the full maturity of their faculties. That assumption is clearly unsupportable in long-term care. For that reason, a thick account of what it means to be a human is required, which would view the range of human autonomy as a corollary of human experience and life and not under pristine theoretical conditions.

One might certainly object that parentalism is nothing more than a semantic sleight of hand because the consequences are the same as weak paternalism, namely, the actions undertaken are not against informed, competent choice, but against encumbered, unreasonable, or incompetent decisionmaking. Perhaps, except for the all-important qualification that weak paternalism typically focuses on the cognitive and volitional capacities that comprise human autonomy whereas parentalism accommodates a broader meaning of autonomy to include affective, conative, and communicative aspects. A consequence of this qualification is the realization that paternalism operates not as direct interference with free action or choice, but insidiously as a latent or tacit feature of the social organization of care that permeates everyday life, not just conflictual decision nodes.

These arguments do not presume to resolve the issue of paternalism. Paternalism has been such a fashionable issue mainly because of two questionable, simplifying assumptions: first, that individuals are by definition (and so in reality) fully capable of rational, free choice and second, that paternalism is as much a compelling concern in everyday life as it is in theory. The first assumption is questionable insofar as it rests on an abstract and somewhat naive view of the reality both of moral life and of decisionmaking or choice. The second assumption is questionable insofar as it is perfectly at home with a thin rather than thick description of the actual phenomena of choice. In many standard discussions of paternalism, autonomy is simply treated entirely in formal or abstract terms due to the general tendency of contemporary ethics to rely on rather weak and contrived examples.

To rectify this situation, it necessary to engage in what Clifford Geertz (1973; 1984) called *thick description*. Ethics would, then, rise to the challenge and find itself at home in those nettlesome complexities of everyday life (Kane and Caplan 1990), rather than in the cloudless and still air of philosophical analysis. As a consequence, ethics would have to become more empirical and phenomenological on the one hand and far more practical and pragmatic on the other. It would require an engagement and involvement in the world of experience that is somewhat lacking even in that growing and motley body of so-called applied ethics. The issue of paternalism as it is so frequently discussed is of interest because it represents an occlusion of a different, and I would suggest a more comprehensive, approach to the ethics of long-term care. Once we see the issue for what it is, we can place paternalism in a wider context of concern, namely, the (sometimes awful) reality of long-term care. The so-called problem of paternalism as a counterpoint to liberty is thus not solved, but rather is transformed from a theoretical puzzle into a practical dialectic animated by what Ronald Dworkin calls concern and respect that together comprise the liberal postulate of equality that takes precedence over liberty as license (1977: 272–73).

Summary

I have argued that liberalism and the liberal view of autonomy are defensible when confined to the political/legal order. Within that realm, autonomy is an indisputably important value, though it may not be the primary value even there. The political/legal realm, however, is not coextensive with human life and certainly does not exhaust the realm of ethics. Primarily, the political/legal concept of autonomy concerns the relationship of individuals and the state and, by extension, the public interactions between strangers in our complex multifaceted society. It only partly defines other aspects of social existence, such as the interactions between intimates of various sorts. Hence, the liberal theory of autonomy and the view of persons that it entails should not be mistaken for an adequate positive account of autonomy. The metaphor of a "realm" clearly needs to be taken with a grain of salt. The image I have in mind is more of overlapping jurisdictions, not closed borders. To use another metaphor, we can confidently say that while the colors of politics and the law are distinct, in actual cases they do bleed into the color of ethics. The important point is that the ways we think about ethics and social relationships need not be reduced to the single dimension of autonomy as negative freedom. Autonomy is a far more complex phenomenon than is routinely appreciated in the standard accounts.

Worries over paternalism naturally flow from a view of autonomy in which independence and noninterference are primary values. Outside the realm of political theory, however, this view proves to be too restrictive. Human beings develop and express their autonomy in a social world. In fact, human beings attain autonomy only through human relationships, particularly relationships with parents. Acknowledging the restrictive nature of the liberal view of autonomy requires that we pay serious attention to human development and human relationships, such as the parent-child relationship. The importance of parenting for understanding human relationships makes it all the more important to distinguish parentalism from paternalism. Doing so helps us to realize that to be autonomous and to exercise one's autonomy requires relations with other persons; at least, then, some of these relationships would support rather than thwart autonomy.

3

Long-Term Care: Myth and Reality

Discussion of autonomy in long-term care is made difficult because assumptions about the nature of caregiving relationships that seem to dominate medical ethics provide inaccurate, inadequate, and misleading norms of long-term care. Long-term care is often assumed to be institutional care in which elders exist without familial or other social supports. It is assumed to involve conflict over basic rights as the "total institution" (Goffman 1960; 1961) strips elders of the vestiges of control and self-respect. The empirical evidence, however, presents a more complicated picture that seems to belie the values of independence and the right of noninterference.

Survey data demonstrate that over 70 percent of home care is delivered by family and friends, not paid providers (Rabin and Stockton 1987: 151). Families contribute financially to the institutional care of older relatives and one in ten younger households is involved in giving care or support to frail older relatives. Rather than the vision of the isolated vulnerable elder in need of the protection afforded by appeal to rights, we find elders sustaining various kinds of integrated lives often in proximity to family and friends. Nonetheless, the received view is that long-term care is predominantly impersonal, institutional, and medical. In this chapter I am concerned less with debunking the mythology associated with being old than in understanding how our thinking about autonomy in long-term care is influenced by cultural prejudices about being old and how this prejudice is reinforced by the dominant model of care in our society based on acute care. To speak of myths is not to speak of false beliefs, since myths are not contrary to reality or truth; instead, myths are deep-seated tacit beliefs that constitute the basic frames of meaning and interpretation in any society.

Myths of Old Age

Simone de Beauvoir noted that the old are invisible because we see death "with a clearer eye" than old age itself (1972: 4). The way elders are perceived by those

47

who are younger and healthier affects the way we behave toward them. Empirical evidence suggests that these modes of perception are socially influenced, if not socially determined. Becoming aware of the mythology and metaphors associated with being old can help us understand the ways that our own interactions with— or avoidances of—elders reflect latent prejudices that need to be exposed if their ethical status is to be assessed.

The effacement of the autonomy of elders takes many forms, but the process of devaluation clearly does not occur in a social vacuum; it is itself a product of assumptions about being old in our society. Uncovering these beliefs and practices is exceedingly difficult. It is sometimes thought that the root of these problems is in institutionalization that inevitably segregates elders from society, but perhaps a truer interpretation is that the phenomenon of nursing home care in America itself reflects diffuse social attitudes and values, though nursing homes undoubtedly contribute to these attitudes in a kind of unrelenting chain reaction. One way to expose the main elements making up the mythology of old age in our society is to review selectively the gerontological literature on the meaning and cultural significance of old age.

A good place to begin is the concept expressed by Rosenfelt under the title "The Elderly Mystique" (1965). Core to the concept of the elderly mystique is the sense that the old person herself explicitly expects derogation. The *elderly mystique* simply holds that the potential for continuing engagement, development, and growth virtually disappears in elders, especially when disabled. A consequence of this mystique is that both professional and other caregivers focus on maintaining activities of daily living and keeping the elderly person out of a nursing home, which encourages the elder to perceive herself as having little or no choice and so experiences a diminished exercise of autonomy (Cohen 1988: 24). It seems to be an outgrowth of an older phenomenon termed by Butler (1975) ageism.

Ageism is a process involving systematic stereotyping of and discrimination against people just because they are old, as racism and sexism does with skin color and gender. Old people are categorized as senile and rigid in thought and manner, and old-fashioned in morality and skills. Ageism allows younger generations to see older people as fundamentally different from themselves, so they subtly cease to identify with their elders as human beings (Butler 1975). Ageism originally described the pejorative cultural attitudes and beliefs about elders that seemed to become a dominant social theme after World War II, though now it appears to be focused less on elders than on elders with disabilities (Cohen 1988: 25). Elders themselves seem to share the view that when a disability arrives hope about growth, self-realization, or participation with family and society must be abandoned so that all energy can be directed toward avoiding "the ultimate defeat, which is not death, but institutionalization which is regarded as a living death" (Cohen 1988: 25).

Richard Taylor (1979) suggested that there is a "new ageism" that is particularly prominent in advocates for elders who stereotypically view all elders in terms of a kind of least common denominator, namely, in terms of those who are least capable, least healthy, and least alert, so that elders as a class are seen as helpless and dependent individuals who require various support services. The development

of these services is encouraged with unbridled enthusiasm and without much concern regarding whether or how these services might reduce the freedom of elders
to make decisions about their own lives. This enthusiasm may be guided by
beneficent motives, but its underlying premise is surely suspect, since the definition of needs and the determination of the kinds of services that adequately meet
these needs are usually made by professionals, not elders themselves. These paternalistic attitudes pose a clear threat to autonomy, especially for disabled and frail
elders who are the most likely recipients of these beneficent intentions and the
least capable of resisting proffered "help."

The negative attitudes toward old age, especially toward disabled elders, is a
corollary of the stress on individualism in the literature on aging, a stress that seems,
in part, a projection of the standards of middle-aged behavior, in which activity
and independence function as tacit norms, onto that of the old. There appears a
latent assumption that successful aging consists in being as much like a middle-
aged person as possible. This means that feeling useful is especially important even
though "feeling useful" has been left undefined. The literature does not make it
clear why old people should be expected to feel that way apparently because the
values of middle age are so tacit (Havighurst 1956: 54–55). If one cannot satisfy
these norms, then that deviance must be explained. The best example of this kind
of explanation is the disengagement theory of aging:

> Starting from the common-sense observation that the old person is less involved
> in the life around him than he was when he was younger, we can describe the
> process by which he becomes so, and we can do this without assumptions about
> its desirability. In our theory, aging is an inevitable mutual withdrawal or disen-
> gagement, resulting in decreased interaction between the aging person and others
> in the social systems he belongs to. His withdrawal may be accompanied at the
> outset by an increased preoccupation with himself; certain institutions in society
> may make this withdrawal easy for him. When the aging process is complete,
> the equilibrium which existed in middle life between the individual and his society
> has given way to a new equilibrium characterized by a greater distance and an
> altered type of relationship. (Cumming and Henry 1961: 14–15)

Thomas Cole (1985) pointed out that in our society a significant gulf separates
age from youth, a gulf that is manifest in the bureaucratized social life course, the
psychological life of individuals, and in the collective imagination of popular culture. When age and youth are fractured into polarities, a self-destructive cycle
evolves. Pointing to progress in the material and physical conditions of life for
elders in the late twentieth century, Americans cannot erase the great spiritual and
ethical price that has been paid. A society that values productivity and material
wealth above other values is understandably youth-oriented; a natural consequence
is that the old come to be seen, and they see themselves, as obsolete and redun-
dant. The cost of such a polarization of youth and old age is significant despite
advances in the material welfare of elders. One cannot conclude that a personally
meaningful sense of security or dignity in old age is attained just because Social
Security and other social programs for the old are in place (Christiansen 1978). In
fact, elders continue to occupy a marginal status in society for the simple reason

that the fundamental social values are wrapped up in a commitment to growth without limit (Cole 1985: 51). As a result, elders are estranged from the main cultural and social forces; they are marginalized not only by the actions of others, actions that might as particular behaviors be quite caring and understanding, but by the value system that makes up our social fabric.

To take elders seriously as full autonomous moral agents, then, must involve more than acknowledging their independence or according them certain rights or entitlements to social services. It means according them full status in the moral community. Beyond invoking the principle of autonomy against professional paternalism or establishing a list of elder rights, understanding the responsibilities or obligations of elders as well as the virtues that age calls for is needed (Jameton 1988; May 1986). Such considerations, however, are seldom prominent concerns. In a sense this is understandable, since the aging industry, including the academic and professional gerontological component, is itself a cultural response to the problem of being old in a society that prizes youth and productivity. Focusing on autonomy as independence follows the common path. Phrasing the problem as a matter of economic, health care, housing, or social service needs has also proved to be enormously popular, while interpreting the problems ethically in terms of the culturally prominent ideal of independence similarly reflects taken-for-granted beliefs. Nevertheless, the fact remains that the underlying paradox or tensions associated with autonomy and long-term care are hardly resolved by such a strategy. For example, the problem of providing adequate health care for our entire population has come up against the social commitments to the aged as a class needing special attention. The resulting problems of setting limits (Callahan 1987) or intergenerational justice (Daniels 1988) are themselves expressions of the underlying cultural confusion about the meaning not only of old age, but of human life itself. The terms of discussion, framed by the liberal model of autonomy, are, like a badly fit suit, not particularly becoming.

Both negative stereotypes of elders as dependent individuals in need of services and incapable of leading "real" lives who are simply an economic drain on society, as well as positive images of elders who are sexually active, healthy, and engaged in their special retirement life-styles reflect a cultural pattern in which elders are generally regarded as outside the social mainstream or culturally disenfranchised (Francher 1969). Perhaps this cultural pattern has been reinforced by the growth of segregated institutions for the aged (Dowd 1985; Gruman 1978), but the deeper question is the symbolic meaning and cultural values that are latent in the isolated status. Importantly, the old represent not only obsolescence and a devalued past, but also a future that no one wants, a future that can be repressed only if the elder is effectively alienated from the vision of one's future self (Cole 1985). The image of the elder as other or stranger is an important cultural development that parallels cultural attitudes about deviants of all sorts who symbolically threaten fundamental beliefs and values central to the individual or social sense of self (Gilman 1988). The earliest visions of the elder as a stranger in the modern period can be found in late eighteenth-century Romantic literature, but it apparently did not become widespread or institutionalized until the growth of retirement (Graebner 1980) and the rise of an industry devoted to aging (Estes 1979). In a sense, efforts to endow elders with a significant social status that they can no longer enjoy in a production and work-oriented society have fostered willy-nilly the meaninglessness and despair that is a commonly observed characteristic of old age.

Negative images of old age in America are sometimes contrasted with other societies. Studies have shown that elders in other societies enjoy considerable respect and occupy important advisory and spiritual roles in family and community, for example, among the Samoans (Holmes and Rhoads 1983), the Druze of Lebanon (Guttman 1976), the Japanese (Plath 1983), the Chinese (Harrell 1979), and many native Americans (Schweitzer 1983). The anthropological evidence, however, is not unequivocal. Other societies such as the Shiriono of Bolivia (Holmberg 1969), the Tasmanians of the South Pacific (Roth 1890), and the Xosa of South Africa (Kidd 1904) are reported to abuse, neglect, or disparage the few old people living in their societies. It would be a mistake to conclude that cultures with more positive attitudes toward elders are the norm and that our society is deviate. The existence of societies that do exhibit positive attitudes and provide positive social roles for their elders supplies us with a set of ideals and shows us what is humanly possible; in doing so, they provide a lens that helps us see what is characteristic of our own society and period in history. "The modern marginality of the old is a hallmark of the very first century to see the elderly become a sizable, problematic portion of the population, with ill-defined roles and responsibilities" (Savishinsky 1991: 2).

The picture of old age in America is thus exceedingly complex because there does not seem to be a single social response to old age and because the meaning of being old is engulfed by cultural beliefs and values that are central to our contemporary social life. Generally, evidence suggests that elders are doing well in retirement despite beliefs held by the medical community and lay people that retirement has an adverse impact on health status (Portnoi 1981). Attitudes among elders toward old age and retirement, such as the images of robustly active retirees normatively projected by groups like the American Association of Retired Persons (AARP), strongly shade the picture. Elders do live in their own homes or apartments, retirement communities, senior citizens' housing complexes, as well as nursing homes. Some are steeped in an ethnic identity and others are devoid of such a heritage. The class of "the elderly" includes both the rich and poor, sick and well, sane and insane; it also embraces the relatively healthy so-called "young old" between sixty and seventy-five and the more vulnerable "old old" who are living beyond their eighth decade. Some are intimately connected to family and community, while others are cut off from their kin. Some are active and ardent; others are disengaged and hopeless (Savishinsky 1991: 2). The picture is probably best described as a collage composed of both complementary and dissonant images. The surest thing to say about old age in America is that it defies easy generalization. Why that is the case is certainly complex, but is rooted in cultural meanings that test and taunt the dominant vision of the person as an isolated, independent, active, and productive individual competently negotiating the everyday world.

Nursing Homes

The mythology of old age in America is important because it is the unavoidable backdrop for any treatment of long-term care. While the causal relations between long-term care and attitudes toward old age in America are speculative at best, there are parallels between the two that help us understand why autonomy is a uniquely relevant problem. As discussed in Chapter 1, long-term care is frequently represented in our society by various icons of nursing home life. These icons of nursing home existence express basic concerns about long-term care that bear directly on the meaning of autonomy itself.

Researchers have identified clear ambiguities and strains in institutional care: for example, some staff think of the institution as a home where others see it as a hospital (Shield 1988); some staff members emphasize humanitarian ideals of care while their colleagues stress cure (Vesperi 1983); and there are pronounced tensions between those who follow a social as opposed to a medical model of treatment (Kane and Kane 1978). One point, however, is clear, namely, that many Americans view old age as joyless and terrible and that nursing homes only make matters worse.

> Such institutions are seen as the last resort of those who can no longer help themselves. In the apparent uselessness of one's later years, they symbolize rejection, and they sometimes rub the salt of neglect into the moral wounds of marginality. This sad, spoiled image of late life contrasts with the equally extreme myth of the golden age of old age, a once hallowed but now suspect truth that people no longer believe in. The imagination of our culture has transformed the old dream into a new nightmare. (Savishinsky 1991: 1)

The overriding theme of most literature on the nursing home experience is one of rejection and loss. In light of this vision of long-term care, one might say of our society what William Butler Yeats said of Byzantium: "That is no country for old men" (1959: 191). The message of much of the literature is that elders, too, find the world of the nursing home quite foreign and forbidding. Unable to manage in the outside world that is inhospitable and unsupportive of their unique needs, they experience the nursing home as a kind of purgatory or limbo, a fate almost worse than death. The titles of some of this literature are remarkably revealing: *A Home is Not a Home* (Tulloch 1975), *Tender Loving Greed* (Mendelson 1975), *Why Survive?* (Butler 1975), *Unloving Care* (Vladeck 1980), *Nobody Ever Died of Old Age* (Curtin 1972), *Old Age: The Last Segregation* (Townsend 1971), *Sans Everything* (Robb 1968), *Uneasy Endings* (Shield 1988), and *The Ends of Time* (Savishinsky 1991).

One of the more personal reports of nursing home life was provided by Carobeth Laird, an anthropologist who at the age of seventy-nine was placed in an Arizona geriatric facility. After her discharge several months later when friends learned of her plight and offered a place to live, she wrote a book entitled *Limbo: A Memoir of Life in a Nursing Home by a Survivor* (1979). She described a number of experiences that are commonly reported for institutionalized elders: a profound loss of control over daily life, an overwhelming sense of isolation, a preoccupation with bodily functions such as eating and excretion, a sense of financial insecurity, a distortion of her own perception of reality and sense of time, and a loss of her sense of self-identity. These are recurrent observations in the nursing home literature that any account of autonomy and the nursing home experience needs to integrate. Although choice was evidently restricted for Laird, loss of choice as such was not the central concern. Other kinds of experience seem to be crucially significant for elders in nursing homes.

Revealing ethnographic work on nursing home life was also done by Maria Vesperi (1983) and Timothy Diamond (1986) who worked as aides in nursing homes. They provide a unique insight into everyday life in nursing homes from the primary caregiver perspective. Nursing assistants constitute one of the largest and fastest growing occupational groups in the United States. Although some men do the work, most nursing assistants are women. As Diamond reported, one of the most important things taught in the training course was not to ask questions or show initiative but to do as one was told. One of the students, a black woman from Jamaica, was reported to joke: "I can't figure out whether they're trying to teach us to be nurses' aides or black women" (1986: 1287). Their daily work is defined mainly in terms of helping elders with sensory and cognitive impairment to complete activities of daily living.

Like the majority of elders in nursing homes, nurses' aides are usually female and often poor (Diamond 1986). They are predominantly nonwhite women even though most owners and directors of nursing homes are white men. Their jobs are hard. Nursing assistants are overwhelmingly paid rates that are scandalously low; hence, the primary providers of care for institutionalized elders are, by any measure, an exploited population. Most nursing assistants are paid at a rate that creates poverty. Even working full-time, they earn less than family subsistence and many assistants are reported to work more than one job if they can or to live in hope of overtime (Diamond 1986: 1288). A society that measures worth and importance largely in monetary terms provides a harsh judgment about the esteem associated with this caregiving. Undoubtedly, this message reverberates in the day-to-day life of the nursing home. For example, as staff turnover occurs, elders are subject to repeated adaptation that introduces a constant source of stress and anxiety into the life of individuals whose coping abilities are compromised by cognitive and physical impairments.

Diamond reported that he brought a number of preconceptions to his work about elders in long-term care. For example, he thought of them as passive recipients of someone else's acts, as acted on rather than acting (1986: 1289). Admittedly, patients are defined by the social structure and organization of nursing homes in a passive way. They are named in terms of their diseases and their basic record of care, the chart, about what is to be done to them, such as feeding, bathing, or toileting, not in terms of what they do. To outside observers it appears a passive existence; infrequent short visits provide snapshot images of people "just sitting" (Diamond 1986: 1289). Day rooms filled with a score of elders are typically bereft of conversation or other apparently meaningful interactions. However, there is another side to the everyday reality of life in a nursing home that evades most casual observers, a reality that extends beyond these static pictures. Once one gets to know elders as individuals, it becomes clear that almost all are thinking and conscious people, though their consciousness might be fragile and intermittent and their concerns different from our own.

Diamond reports that elders actively participate in various nursing home settings. They are not simply acted on but struggle to maintain their own consciousness and identity, even if appearances belie this effort (Diamond 1986: 1290). If appearances belie this effort, it is because we assume that real work is objectified in the world as a "work," a material object produced by one's efforts. Work is closely related to the phenomena of pain and imagination; like them it presses toward objectification, though the objectification is not always so evidently a physical thing in the world (Scarry 1985). Rather, the work activities in which many (particularly institutionalized) elders engage involves remaking the world for experience, reconstituting the meaning structures for their lives, not simply forming objects within the ambient world. Too often, the kind of effort required for such world-making is overlooked because standard accounts of autonomy never adequately address the need for individuals to actively define or make a world, focusing instead on discrete choices or decisions within a pregiven frame of reality or reference. The clear implication of these points is that any adequate account of autonomy in long-term care needs to understand and make sense of the activity of world-making in which even seemingly passive or confused elders unavoidably engage.

Although nursing home residents are not by definition passive, they are remarkably dependent. The ability to perform activities of daily living such as dressing and grooming, bathing or eating cannot safely be assumed for these individuals. In fact, the job description of nurses' aides most involves performing the basic functions of daily living such as helping individuals get in and out of bed, giving baths, assisting elders in the toilet or in feeding. The 1985 National Nursing Home Survey reports that 91 percent of residents needed help with bathing, 75 percent with dressing, 63 percent with getting in and out of bed or a chair, 40 percent with eating, and 50 percent experienced some bladder or bowel incontinence (Hing 1987).

Coupled with the need for assistance in routine activities of daily living, most elders in nursing homes suffer from various sensory and cognitive impairments: for example, 63 percent of all nursing home residents are demented or have serious memory impairments (Hing 1987). Although some caution is in order in interpreting this data, since the diagnostic data are dependent on a notation in the chart that normally was the result of an assumption rather than a serious work up (Kane 1990: 9), considerable cognitive impairment undoubtedly exists in nursing homes. Some studies indicate that as many as 75 percent of nursing home residents have some mental impairment (Larsen, Lo, and Williams 1986). These data, however, do not necessarily mean that autonomy is absent, though prejudices associated with mental illness commonly assume that anyone who is mentally ill or mentally impaired is by definition incompetent. These facts cannot be overlooked in conceptualizing autonomy in long-term care. Other findings, too, are relevant. For example, after surveying 111 programs in a three-state area, Hegeman and Tobin (1988) reported that the functioning of mentally impaired elders can be improved by a diversity of interventions including special programming such as small group activities involving reminiscence, validation therapy, discussion, and sensory stimulation; structural and environmental adaptations; and staff training and deployment. Even some of the most confused residents can be helped to preserve their remaining identity and disorganized incompetent elders can be helped to be more oriented to time and place, thus providing them with some of the prerequisites for self-determination.

Studies of nursing homes, however, are rife with evidence that various common practices infantilize and depersonalize elders, including loss of privacy, restrictions on having personal possessions or the ability to entertain guests, and the unavailability of transportation or in-house services. Coupled with the need to adapt to the "total" environment of a nursing home that isolates, controls, and reconstitutes the daily lives of elders who live in them, these practices constitute impressive assaults on autonomy. Since staff are primarily oriented toward pursuing medically related activities—the dominant mode of discourse, the schedule, and work evaluations are based on the performance of such specific tasks as bathing, feeding, or toilet assistance—the full effect of this orientation for the autonomy of elders goes unnoticed. The medically defined objectives rarely take into account the elder as an experiencing subject and person who is the object of this care.

Vesperi (1983) noted a fundamental contradiction between patient expectations and staff goals. The predominant training model for nurses' aides is a medical model. The education of nurses' aides and their daily work is defined in a task-centered physical way (Diamond 1986: 1290). The day starts with staff members having to rouse patients who invariably grumble at the early awakening times. Elders must awaken, get dressed, and get prepared for breakfast and medications. They are then transported, if not bedfast, to the day room for breakfast. If the nurse's aide is stuck with too many "feeders," namely, patients who need help eating, it could prove impossible to finish breakfast at the appointed time. Coupling the slow pace of many elders in eating, particularly those who dislike the food or are still not yet fully awake and alert, with the relentless rush of the scheduled close of breakfast, staff naturally feel anxious and hardly relaxed to engage in any kind of meaningful interaction with their charges. After breakfast activities, such as helping elders with showers or bed baths, toileting or bed pans, changing beds, taking vital signs, and responding to continuous individual requests, and recording it all in the chart, keep the staff extremely busy until lunch when the ordeal of the meal resumes.

Much of this activity is important and essential in the care of institutionalized elders, though it is often infused with meanings that are bizarre at best. Despite all the attention to physical well-being and the maintenance of the trappings of the hospital, such as uniforms, charts, and recording vital signs, there is little real therapeutic intent. The treatment simply does not work toward this objective, but is carried out at the level of custodial care. As Savishinsky reported, "this lack of emphasis on restoring people's health defeated the best hopes of residents and intensified their tendency to decline" (1991: 6). The underlying problem is not only the way that restoring health or maintaining well-being is pursued, but unclarity or controversy regarding the basic meaning of health or well-being for an institutionalized frail elder.

Even though nursing homes are not hospitals, they are medical environments. The trappings of the hospital are in evidence everywhere from the chart, recording the units of health care one receives, and the diagnosis or sickness category, to the spotless, sanitized environment and the officiously busy, uniformed staff. Daily work is defined in a task-centered fashion focused on provision of services associated with activities of daily living. Task responsibility is oriented toward the objective action to be performed rather than the recipient of the action (Agich 1982: 66). It thrives in a bureaucratic organization in which the hierarchical structure of authority promotes an external accountability for one's behavior rather than a subjective or internal accountability in terms of one's own judgment. This understanding of the basic caregiver's responsibility contributes to the feeling of estrangement and frustration that nurses' aides reportedly exhibit. The bureaucratic structure of the typical nursing home assures that supervisory staff, who are usually found to be well-removed from the actual caregiving, have little actual appreciation of what it takes for nurses' aides to accomplish daily work routines and how the structure of daily work effectively thwarts any vestiges of autonomy. Coupled with the low levels of pay, education, and undeniable stress of work, direct-care staff understandably display negative work attitudes as evidenced by the high rate at which they resign (Diamond 1986: 1287–88; Savishinsky 1991: 5).

Although the nursing home is commonly viewed as a way station on the road to death, national data suggest a more complicated picture. There is good reason to assume that there are two separate streams of patients passing through nursing homes: a short-stay group whose average length of stay is approximately 1.9 months and a long-stay group who stay about 2.5 years. Although the latter accounts for only 39 percent of discharges, they comprise 91 percent of the residents at any one time (Keeler, Kane, and Solomon 1981). Taking into account all nursing home residents, the average length of stay was about one year, though some residents stayed for decades. Although nursing homes are prominent sites of long-term care for many elders, they are remarkably transient institutions. There is considerable coming and going as patients are discharged, reassigned to different units based on staff judgments about (among other things) the level and kind of care needed, and new ones admitted. Coupled with staff turnover, an air of confusion, unreality, and rootlessness naturally emerges. Despite the amount and significance of change for residents, they typically have little or no say except for feeble protest.

The make-up of nursing homes inevitably includes individuals with diverse interests, backgrounds, social and educational class, former occupations, and income (Macklin 1990). They are anything but communities or homes; little or nothing is done to foster, or even to permit, meaningful relationships or associations to develop. Indeed, assignment of roommates or rooms, a commonplace occurrence in nursing homes, poses significant ethical questions that have only recently been the subject of ethical analysis (Miles and Sachs 1990).

Institutions that are church-run or have a distinct ethnic or religious make-up surprisingly show the same anomie and meaningless characteristic of secular institutions. Jaber Gubrium (1975) observed that day-to-day routines centered on the cognitive organization of life and labor of a church-run institution he called Murray Manor. He described various structural divisions between "top staff" and "floor staff," the nature and conduct of "bed and body" work by floor staff, the ritual outings of residents and the unique status enjoyed by those who received visitors, and the implicit and explicit ways that elders staked out personal space by claiming chairs or lounge areas. Gubrium reported that an ethic of sensitive individualized care was propounded by administrators who were comfortably removed from the everyday work world of floor staff so that they infrequently saw how patients were actually treated.

Mary O'Brien (1989) described Bethany Manor, a 230-bed east coast nursing home whose funding, supervisory staff, and elders were primarily drawn from the local Catholic community. The facility's religious atmosphere and services did seem to help many residents develop and sustain an accepting attitude toward death, but this did not mean that all anxieties and fears associated with being old and frail were absent. There was, for instance, a significant fear of surviving with a lingering cognitive deficit (O'Brien 1989: 96) or being transferred to the third floor, a fate that was viewed singly worse than death (O'Brien 1989: 32).

Renée Rose Shield (1988) similarly described a nonprofit Jewish facility located in a northeastern city. While residents shared a common religious background, the facility was not able to provide them with a sense of community or any effectively meaningful way to ease their transition to old age and impairment. Shield attributed these deficiencies to several factors including the controlling nature of the institutional regulations, the inability of elders to reciprocate what others gave them, the tendency of elders to preserve their autonomy by remaining aloof one from another, and a lack of staff consensus regarding whether the facility was a home or a hospital. As a result, various inequities and contradictions were expressed in institutional rules that tended to place residents and staff in adversarial relationships (Shield 1988: 22).

The picture of long-term care presented in the nursing home literature is clearly bleak. This situation is in part attributable to the way the United States funds long-term care as a health-related "welfare" benefit for the poor rather than a health benefit or social service for all. It is a matter of public policy that long-term care benefits depend on medical definitions of "need for care" (Kane and Kane 1990: 86). Ironically, the more dependent people are, the more eligible they are for care based on their inability to perform specific basic activities such as ADL (activities of daily living) and IADL (instrumental activities of daily living). The result is a payment system that rewards dependency by creating disincentives to caregivers to help clients recover or improve functioning; by definition, this payment system impedes or thwarts autonomy (Kane and Kane 1990: 86).

Part of the difficulty is the emphasis given to formal rehabilitation services that have as their goal maximizing the functional abilities of disabled and impaired elders over other care that is viewed as merely custodial. Unless elders are formally eligible for a reimbursable rehabilitation program, they are not usually helped to improve their functioning. As a result, payment mechanisms limit areas of choice about the place and type of care as well as constrain many daily choices that elders make. Ironically, elders with functional impairments require the help of others to carry out their choices, so that autonomy may actually be restricted precisely when an elder's independence is "respected." When elders require help to do things for themselves but that help is not available for reimbursement or bureaucratic reasons, positive autonomy is existentially compromised.

This point involves the distinction between decisional and executional autonomy (Collopy 1988). *Decisional autonomy* is the ability to make decisions without external restraint or coercion. *Executional autonomy* is the ability and freedom to act on decisional autonomy. For most individuals, autonomy is both decisional and executional, but it need not always be so and individuals can be able to decide, while lacking the ability or freedom to execute decisions. An implication of this distinction is that if autonomy is defined primarily by execution, then frail and confused elders will be by definition nonautonomous. However, because decisional autonomy can remain intact when executional autonomy wanes, failure to provide adequate help to an incapacitated elder can seriously efface autonomy. As Collopy noted, "as the outward reach of autonomy shrinks, its inner decisional core becomes a last and therefore most crucial preserve of self-determination" (1988: 12). Supporting executional autonomy, then, is an important way to respect overall an elder's autonomy. Doing so, however, entails more than simply forbearance because specific help or services need to be positively provided.

Present nursing home reimbursement is perverse because it is focused on estimates of time required by various personnel to care for particular types of elders. The result is that the more an elder needs help with activities of daily living, exhibits behavioral problems, or requires more nursing procedures, the more the institution is reimbursed. Dependent elders are thus more valuable, from a reimbursement standpoint, than more functional elders. The result of these incentives is that "enthusiasm for making residents less dependent is muted" (Kane and Kane 1990: 87). Time spent motivating and instructing elders is excluded from the calculations, a fact that has not escaped astute administrators. Because reimbursement is determined on the basis of the efficient provision of specific, discrete services, not overall improvement in the quality of care or life of the elder, interactions become routinized. In effect, the entire atmosphere is regimented and mechanized. In part, this is understandable given the "production" mentality of the medical model that strongly influences the provision of care for elders. It is small consolation that things are not much better with home care. The payment system reimburses only those providers who have been formally certified by regulatory agencies. Hence, elders are basically prevented from recruiting their own help. A defender of negative freedom might, of course, object that elders are not forced to forego hiring help of their own choosing, provided that they can pay for it. When ability to pay is limited, then benefits that constrain choice in ways that are undesirable for elders does seem to violate the positive requirements of autonomy. If enhancement or preservation of autonomy is a goal of long-term care, then restricting choice by regulation can adversely impact autonomy.

Medicare does not provide reimbursement for things needed to maintain independent functioning such as transportation away from the nursing home. Institutionalized elders are thus unable to freely visit families, pursue their own chosen activities, or develop their own schedules. Effectively, they are incarcerated in the institution in which they live. Empirical work has shown striking dissonance between preferences expressed by the elders and those acknowledged by staff.

Elders rate trips out of the facility and the use of the telephone as very important, whereas staff most often thought that organized nursing home activities such as bingo or arts and crafts were most important and least often thought that using the telephone was important at all (Kane, Freeman, *et al.* 1990: 70).

One conclusion that could be drawn from these observations is that nursing homes simply need reform. Guided by the ideal of autonomy as independence, institutionalized elders need to be set free, liberated. Liberation is unquestionably an appropriate implication of a concern for autonomy in long-term care, but one should scrupulously inquire into the actual conditions requisite for liberation. For colonial states, liberation is a justifiable political goal, but achieving that goal does not guarantee the economic sufficiency necessary for true state sovereignty. Analogously, liberation for elders in nursing homes is far too simplistic a solution if it follows the political tack of providing independence alone. Similarly, reforms that focus on the institutional structure or on specific problems without an adequate framework supporting a positive view of autonomy are likely to prove ineffectual because something more subtle and insidious is involved.

Latent generalizations about what it is to be old in our society form a sedimentary layer that needs excavation and evaluation. Attitudes and beliefs that underlie explanations of the behavior of elders such as "that's the way they are when they're old" (Shield 1988: 16) involve treating elders abstractly, as members of a category rather than as individuals. In a sense, elders seldom are seen as "us," but as somehow fundamentally different and alien. Regarding elders as Other is an example of a wider phenomenon of treating as alien things that constitute a fundamental threat to our own sense of self or well-being (Gilman 1988). This behavior can be confronted not by simply insisting that autonomy be respected, but by probing further into the seminal meanings to which nursing home care seems committed.

One concept to which nursing homes are stalwartly committed is that of the therapeutic relationship. Although there is some disagreement over whether a social or medical approach is best in the management of particular cases or as a philosophy for a particular institution, the overall model is therapeutic. With the therapeutic model, however, comes powerful expectations such as "following doctor's orders" that effectively shape, and some would say inhibit, the style and substance of interactions. To appreciate the effect this might have on autonomy, it is worthwhile considering the expectations generally associated with the concept of the therapeutic in contemporary society.

Therapeutic Relationships

A *therapeutic relationship* is a relationship between an individual who suffers some defect, disability, or discomfort and a practitioner who possesses a specific technical skill or knowledge and who occupies a recognized social role. The primary goal of the relationship is to improve the well-being of the suffering individual as the result of action that is undertaken within the relationship. It is no wonder, then, that professional medical ethics is frequently described as an agency ethic (American College of Physicians 1984b: 266; Beauchamp and Childress 1983: 213; Daniels 1986: 1382; Fried 1978: 243; Pellegrino and Thomasma 1981: 275), that is, an ethic in which the practitioner is obligated to function as the agent of the patient acting in the patient's best interest as determined by professional judgment. Although this ethic seems paternalistic, there are important considerations that support carefully distinguishing paternalism and beneficence in medicine as discussed in Chapter 2. For present purposes, it is important to note that the definition of well-being pursued and the judgments made regarding the presenting problem (the defect, deficiency, or disability) are interrelated in complex ways that require reference to the practice in which the therapeutic relationship is a constituent part (Agich 1983b).

Therapeutic relationships exhibit three general interdependent features: a particular structure and style of interaction, a particular intention to improve or contribute to the well-being of an individual (as well as a particular definition or understanding of what constitutes sickness and well-being), and a particular set of techniques or skills that are possessed and exercised by the practitioner that can broadly be referred to as therapy. It is thus assumed or required that possession of expert knowledge, skill, or technique is an essential feature of being a practitioner. As a corollary, practitioners acquire a special power over patients, a power that naturally gives rise to concerns about paternalism.

The definition just offered defines the essential features of therapeutic relationships *in general*. Individual kinds of therapeutic relationships exhibit these features in different ways. By focusing on the kinds of skill, techniques, or interactions that are possible and the correlative definitions of the well-being sought, one can develop a taxonomy of therapeutic relationships. Historically, not only medicine and health care, but philosophy, religion, and art were seen as therapeutic. In contemporary America the dominant understanding of the therapeutic is based on the sick role as represented in acute care medicine. This model involves an asymmetrical relationship between the sick person and therapeutic agencies.

The *sick role* has three primary elements: first, the acceptance by both self and others that being ill is not the sick person's fault and that she should be seen as a victim of forces beyond her control; second, there is a claimed exemption from usual daily expectations and obligations; and third, if the illness is sufficiently severe, then the sick person will seek help from some health care provider (Parsons 1975: 262). The sick role concept captures the predominant social model of illness in our society. To understand the way the sick role influences our thinking about autonomy in long-term care requires reflecting on how therapeutic relationships are modeled in the practice of medicine.

The therapeutic practice itself primarily contributes to defining the nature of well-being as well as shaping judgments about disability or disease, rather than just treating the ill individual. This is important. I argue in Chapter 4 that identification with beliefs, choices, and values that are truly one's own is logically prior to freedom and is the core element in autonomy of persons. If this argument is sound, then the fact that the experience and perception of individuals fails to correspond with that of society and practitioners does not just create occasions for conflict that activates concern for autonomy as negative freedom, but autonomy is at stake at the more basic level of underlying belief and value. Alienation of the ill individual from the socially defined sick role and the meanings associated with the disease diagnosis is thus not only possible, but inevitable. This fact poses important ethical questions. Human existence is essentially social, yet the autonomy of persons involves identifications that can creatively depart from social norms and expectations. Tensions, if not contradictions, are therefore unavoidable. An approach that can constructively deal with these not only as quandaries or problems to be resolved, but as involving basic questions of virtue and character is sorely needed (May 1986).

Philip Rieff discussed the striking difference between what he termed *classical* (or traditional) and *modern* views of therapy (1966). Modern views of therapy are primarily concerned with "what cures." Classical views are concerned with "who cures." On the classical view it is ultimately the community that cures because the function of the classical therapist is to commit the patient to the symbol system of the community by means of those techniques sanctioned by the community, for example, ritual, dialectical, magical, or rational. As Rieff put it:

> All such efforts to reintegrate the subject into the community symbol system may be categorized as "commitment therapies." Behind shaman and priest, philosopher and physician stems the great community as the ultimate corrective of personal disorders. (1966: 68–69)

Modern views of therapy, however, function where the community itself is disordered and not able to supply a system of symbolic integration. As a result, the therapeutic function of the community is either absent or compromised; instead, it is transferred to a special group of individuals who treat individual patients as individuals, not community representatives who reintegrate the sick person into the community. An implication of this changed view of therapy is that caregiving, too, is transformed from an activity that is readily available and possibly disseminated within the community to an activity that is separate and apart from everyday life surrounded by a special professional aura. Shamans certainly carry with them a special aura, yet their function is open to the community in the sense that it expresses deeply held and widely shared beliefs. Mystery, of course, surrounds a good deal of the therapeutic proceedings, but it is attached to the community and the sick individual by a shared worldview in which the nature and meaning of sickness is continuous with everyday experience. In the modern world that is not the case.

Despite cultural faith in scientific progress, the central meanings of the biomedical and clinical sciences are hardly continuous with everyday experience and structures of explanation. One important result is the way that there is dissonance between patient and physician understandings of illness. This dislocation or separation creates a different kind of mystery and a different kind of power for the modern physician when compared with traditional healers. The sick individual is, by virtue of the sickness, literally a patient and is thus different from others, especially the physician, whose agency is still fully intact. Patients are simply expected to take their medicine; it is not necessary that the patient's view of illness accord with the physician's understanding. The main requirement is compliance with doctor's orders, but that is mostly a matter of performance or a willingness to undergo the physician's interventions, not a matter of the patient's personal belief.

The power of modern medicine rests on its causal efficaciousness without the need for a concordance of belief between healer and patient. As a result, in the modern concept of the therapeutic, truth is displaced as a value. The patient does not need to believe, understand, or know because modern medicine operates outside the sphere of communal or personal validation. The modern concept of the therapeutic thus has little need for widespread social understanding or support, relying instead on a narrower and specialized scientific standard of truth. Of course, one might object that this scientific standard of truth is itself socially accepted, but the acceptance seems predicated on a global and mostly blind faith in scientific progress and technology, not on an understanding of even key scientific concepts and commitments. The acceptance of science is predicated less on the meaningful way that it explains common social experience than on its power as technology (Agich 1981). There exists a striking gap between scientific and everyday modes of explanation.

Since the therapeutic has become appropriated as a concept of specialized, professional knowledge, the sick person is conceived to be without resources to help herself. This means that autonomy is by definition waived or compromised by illness on this view. The sick individual becomes fully a patient and so ceases to be an agent (MacIntyre 1977). In this regard it is enlightening to note that informed consent is a uniquely modern development. Not only does informed consent reflect the prominence of individual self-determination, but it functions precisely in a social context in which solidarity or commitment to a basic belief system is rare. To be a therapist to individuals, who are independent and isolated from a wider community of meaning, thus requires that the therapist be similarly severed or disconnected from the community at large. The predictable result is that not binding sentiment, but critical detachment becomes the attitude most conducive to a sense of well-being on the modern view (MacIntyre 1981: 29; cf. Koch 1972).

Concepts of health and disease may be defined in terms of consensus regarding values and beliefs, but cure or successful therapy may not be achievable simply by the power of consensus or public opinion. There are obvious limits to the power of consensus to correct or ameliorate serious defects, disabilities, or discomforts. One cannot rationally expect that even widely shared beliefs will prevent or cure disease or correct disabilities or discomforts because the relation of beliefs to effective action is not logical, but empirical. In other words, simply because one believes that a secret potion obtained through mail order and highly recommended by friends will cure arthritis does not assure a cure. This point is true enough, but perhaps its usefulness is limited; if informed consent is important, then what individuals believe in and value, even what is therapeutically efficacious, must be taken into account by health care providers. Interestingly, this point has been made in prominent medical journals, for example, by Lidz, Appelbaum, and Meisel (1988) as one of the phases of patient care that establishes a "process" model of informed consent and by Pankratz and Kofoed (1988) as a recommendation for assessing and treating "geezers." That social role and causal effectiveness can be separated is shown by the fact that people may be able to heal or actually suffer independently of the opinion of their society (Neu 1975: 112).

The distinction between modern and classical views of therapy and the therapeutic relationship would be misleading if it were taken either to indicate that medicine, and particularly the modern physician-patient relationship, are not supported by social consensus or that therapeutic power is simply a direct result of social consensus. The actual case seems to contradict both of these conclusions. The way that medicine provides the dominant model for long-term care, however, involves assumptions that support an individualistic view of therapy and a concept of the causal effectiveness of therapeutic interventions that are radically different from the classical view described by Rieff. The implications of this distinction can be made clear by focusing on the nature of illness and disease in our society.

Concepts of Illness and Disease

In modern medicine, illness or disease is not defined positively, but privatively in terms of an inability to exercise rational free agency (Engelhardt 1976). This may be due either to the absence of social consensus regarding a positive definition of human well-being or it may be due to a recognition of the empirical and fallible character of diagnosis. In any event, the negative definition of well-being or health in terms of disease categories appears to be primary in contemporary medicine. Thus, those conditions or states of affairs that reduce or restrict rational free action tend to count as diseases; those states that augment rational free action count as health (Engelhardt 1976).

One implication of this view is that concepts of health and disease are "plastic" because rational free agency is an abstract concept that can be specified in many ways. What counts as a disease thus depends in large part on what suffering human beings as finite rational agents are willing to accept and on the kind of lives they wish to live. These judgments are not the product of idiosyncratic preference, however, but reflect a general, social view predominant at certain historical periods regarding what contributes to or thwarts rational free agency. Consensus is involved but consensus concerns certain abstract or general values and norms whose specification is left to the practice of medicine as a historical and empirical enterprise. In this practice, the availability of scientific and empirical techniques for intervening in and altering those states or conditions that compromise free action figures importantly in defining what counts as a disease as well as for legitimating illness.

Since autonomy is understood on this model abstractly, anything that restricts rational free agency tends to count as disease. As a consequence, aging itself can be seen as a disease, as something disvalued, because it entails a restriction on rational free action (Caplan 1984; Engelhardt 1979). Thus, not only do elders suffer from diseases that are shared with younger members of society, they also can be seen to suffer from a pervasive disease of a long life, namely, being old. Such a notion of disease evidently despises dependence above all else. Dependence due to disability or frailty constitutes a fundamental judgment of the disvalue of elders, particularly those who are impaired as occurs under the newer versions of "the elderly mystique" (Cohen 1988).

The impact of this model on long-term care is significant. First, the model reinforces existing social values regarding the aversion for dependency and the preference for independence above all else. Medical treatment is seen as interference and is tolerated only insofar as it aims at (and achieves) cure. Treatment, in other words, is tolerated insofar as it is able to return the individual to the pre-existing state of independent and competent free agency. Such a goal, however, seems both inappropriate and cruel in long-term care. It sets expectations that because they cannot be met, seem to encourage caregivers to offer less care or to accept the inevitability of dependence. It is no wonder then that long-term care focuses on "bed and body" work and the person who is the subject of such work is forgotten. It is as if the elder ceased to exist once it became clear that ideal independence could not be restored. The notion of a therapeutic environment for the impaired or frail elder will not likely be established on the conceptual basis of contemporary medicine since it fundamentally disvalues not only the illnesses of elders, but their very existential status as old and frail.

Models of Care

One difficulty that confronts discussion of the problem of autonomy in long-term care is that medical ethics, like medicine itself, is acute care and in-patient oriented. Typically, a patient is institutionalized for short periods of time for discrete problems: the majority of care is provided by cadres of health professionals who usually have brief, procedure or task-oriented encounters with the patient. Clinical decisionmaking, too, typically has a short time horizon: the goal is improvement of biological status to the point that permits discharge. Discharge is usually predicated on removal from the unit, not necessarily discharge from the hospital. The goal of resuming normal activities or regaining a premorbid quality of experience and range of activities is hardly ever explicitly the main object of concern for health professionals, though for patient and family these are typically the preoccupation. Restoration of normal ABGs (arterial blood gases), for example, is a primary goal for pulmonologists and nurses in pulmonary and intensive care units, but it is rare for these scores to be related in any meaningful way to the patient's future life-style except, and only until, they are normalized or therapeutic defeat is acknowledged. The orientation is thus exceedingly short term, problem-defined, and task-dominated. Bureaucratic organization of the delivery of services further exacerbates the alienation of health professionals from the patient as a person.

Given the dominance of the acute care orientation in American medicine, it is not at all surprising that bioethical thinking has come to focus on the paradigm cases and problems that arise in acute care medical settings. This focus is usually marked by crisis and conflict; ethics becomes relevant only when all else fails because the basic orientation is on specific problems, procedures, and tasks. Given the structural features of the way health care is delivered, conflict is inevitable.

Conflict arises under conditions of great stress and under circumstances that do not afford sufficient opportunity to ameliorate disagreement. It is no wonder, then, that rights language has come to dominate medical ethics. Profoundly influenced by medical-legal developments, medical ethics has wholly adopted, and certainly adapted, concepts such as informed consent that had their origin in the malpractice arena (Faden and Beauchamp 1986). The consequence is that legalism is a dominant feature of medical ethics, which helps explain why medical ethics tends to focus on conflictual and dramatic problems and relies heavily on the language of rights instead of, for example, the language of responsibility (Agich 1982; Ladd 1978).

Conflict is also inevitable because of the fundamental orientation of acute medical care toward patient welfare as judged by the physician. Beneficence dominates this model. It is accepted because the disruption posed by sickness or illness is usually well-defined and reversible. The physician can arrive at relatively unambiguous determinations of patient need and reliable assessments of the risks and benefits associated with proposed or alternate therapies. Informed consent, or better still, informed choice, involves presenting patients with an array of options that are discrete and readily understandable. Patient needs as well as the risks and benefits associated with treatment are defined for the patient by the physician. In long-term care, however, the principle of beneficence is less powerful and so affords a weaker basis for caregiver authority. One reason this principle is less dominant is because physicians are usually only remotely involved in long-term care and then usually at some distance from day-to-day treatment. As a result, autonomy becomes not only more important, but takes on positive features lacking in the acute care-based medical model that supports simple informed choice.

Elders who need long-term care suffer from chronic conditions that are not curable. Risks and benefits cannot be readily ascertained and, in any event, clearly involve elements that are not necessarily excluded by the much more diffuse model of long-term care. For example, the sick role concept underlying acute medical care assumes that the sick person will cooperate with health professionals to restore premorbid functioning, indeed, has the obligation to do so. Long-term care, by definition, precludes a return to premorbid, normal functioning, so personal or idiosyncratic considerations that would otherwise be trumped by the obligation to get well retain their validity. Long-term care needs also tend to involve multiple, overlapping physical, psychological, and social dimensions that cannot all be readily conceptualized, much less managed, in strict medical terms (Hofland 1988: 5).

Even for clear medical needs there is often greater uncertainty and a wider range of possible interventions. Because the goal cannot be cure, the diagnostic and therapeutic certainty of the acute care model finds little to grip. Lacking the traction provided by the goal of curing as the main ingredient of patient welfare, patient preferences and values become far more important. In the acute care context, especially in hospitals, patients are intimidated by the foreign environment. In contrast, home care is delivered on the patient's own turf and institutional care occurs where the patient resides, so patient autonomy is in a more fertile environment. Despite these "environmental" differences, long-term care, especially nursing home care, seems to efface rather than enhance the residual autonomy of elders.

The nursing home mystique exerts a subtle and pervasive influence on thinking about long-term care. Largely because of the migration of the medical model into the nursing home, the emphasis is on medical or nursing care even though there seems to be little such care actually given. Typically, nursing homes are structured in form and circumstance very much like hospitals: physical arrangement of rooms, furniture, maintenance of records, distribution of medications, presence of a "nursing station" even though most care is provided by aides rather than trained nurses. These structural elements affect the everyday practice of caregiving in nursing homes; collectively, they convey powerful expectations about who the elder is and what is the elder's proper role. This is evident in the way that the medical condition of individuals who live in nursing homes tends to dominate much of the formal structure as well as day-to-day activity (Gubrium 1975; Lidz, Fischer, and Arnold 1990; Savishinsky 1991; Shield 1988). Elders are referred to by their medical condition, their unit or room number, or simply as "that patient" (Lidz, Fischer, and Arnold 1990: 69–86). Elders seem no more differentiating about staff than staff are about elders. In their ethnographic study of autonomy in long-term care, Lidz, Fischer, and Arnold, reported that in spite of considerable efforts at explanation, their female observer was sometimes called "nurse" even though she wore street clothes and provided no nursing care. Patients seemed either unable or disinterested in making any distinctions between the different staff members who cared for them (1990: 69–70).

The history and sociology of nursing homes are part of a larger phenomenon—the institutionalization of social deviants, such as criminals, indigents, the insane, and orphans. Rothman (1971) convincingly argued that the trend toward institutionalization in the United States was mainly an attempt to deal with a wide range of problems, such as crime, poverty, and severe illness, that were seen for the first time as social in nature. Institutions were seen as serving both preventive and rehabilitative purposes, particularly in Jacksonian America, and were developed on the basis of principles and routine. Programs were designed to separate the aged, chronically ill, and disabled from those able to work to allow each institution to impose a special routine on its particular population. This heritage of regimentation and social engineering is evident in nursing homes today. It is, however, mediated by the development of specific medical institutions like the acute care hospital that has exerted such a profound influence on the structure of American medicine and medical ethics and is supported by a payment system that rewards efficiency in the provision of specific services, but not necessarily care of elders as such (Kane and Kane 1990).

The federal regulation of nursing homes involves two major sets of regulatory requirements. One contains the requirements that facilities must meet to participate in Medicare and Medicaid (Code of Federal Regulations 1987a; 1987b). The second covers the enforcement process that the federal government and its agents, namely, the state survey agencies, must follow in inspecting nursing homes and approving or disapproving them for participation (Code of Federal Regulations 1987c). When this process began in 1965 with the passage of Medicare, long-term care facilities presented special problems because no regulatory model existed for either skilled or intermediate care facilities. The Joint Commission hospital or medical model did exist and that model was adapted to derive a new set of regulations for nursing homes (Morford 1988: 129).

Two concerns dominated these regulations: safety and adequacy of treatment and services. Addressing physical safety was relatively straightforward. The facilities should be fire safe and clean and staff should not abuse patients. These concerns are the so-called bricks and mortar requirements that historically prompted major improvements in America's nursing homes because fire, filth, and patient abuse were not uncommon problems. Adequacy of treatment and services, however, was not a concern easily addressed. One simply cannot mandate good results, as such regulations would amount to little more than desiderata, not measurable and enforceable guidelines. Instead, the measures adopted took the form of spelling out enforceable policies, procedures, and qualifications that were assumed to stand in for outcome.

One cannot, for example, assure that successful surgery will occur in hospitals simply by mandating success in surgery, but one can try to promote that outcome by requiring surgeons to meet specific qualifications or follow appropriate procedures and policies. In nursing homes, the same principles were applied; detailed policies, procedures, and qualifications were promulgated in lieu of direct outcome measures (Morford 1988: 129). There is reason to believe that these standards are actually outcome insensitive. Whether that is true or not is a complicated question, but it does seem evident that these standards are not particularly sensitive to promoting or maintaining autonomy in nursing home residents (Kane and Kane 1990). In fact, the burdens of complying with the standards, such as meeting recordkeeping requirements, divert scarce staff time and effort from other activities. The overriding problem is that the nursing home regulations impose a task-oriented medical model of care on what might be better thought of in other terms.

The Concept of a Practice

To explore the impact of acute care medicine on the understanding of autonomy in medical ethics, it is useful to reflect on the similarities and differences between acute care medicine and long-term care as practices by considering first the defining features of a practice. Two general features of practices are important (Flathman 1976; 1980). The first is the rule-governed character of practices. A practice can be defined as a set of ordered activities that is characterized by patterns of regularity. The term *rule* refers not only to the seeming "objective" regularities that can be observed in the behaviors of participants in a practice and are catalogued by social scientists, but also to the regularities and norms that define the practice for the participants and that participants in the practice knowingly and intentionally follow. In this sense, rules are less like objective laws of nature providing explanatory frameworks than they are like rules of thumb or recipes for action that all social actors, including social scientists, employ in engaging in particular practices.

The rules of a practice include the specialized knowledge, skills-at-hand, and procedures that normatively define the status of individuals as practitioners or as participants in the practice in question. Following rules and knowing which rules to follow is one feature that defines individuals as participants in a practice. This is not simply an abstract requirement, but reflects actual experience. Behaviors and organizational structures associated with nursing homes discussed above, such as taking vital signs, charting care activities performed for patients, and bureaucratic organization, reflect rules derived from hospital-based care. To function as a caregiver in a nursing home involves learning a wide-range of rules that are task-oriented, geared toward helping elders to complete basic activities of daily living.

The rules of a practice, however, are not free standing. They depend on a logically distinct but related set of values and beliefs that provide participants a basis for accepting and following rules. Rules guide conduct only where there is acceptance of ways of thinking and acting that have a wider significance and relevance than the particular rules themselves. In other words, rules must "make sense" socially, they must afford a basis for meaningful social action. What constitutes "meaningful" social action is determined in part by reference to values and beliefs of the participants. It is these values and beliefs that provide the basis on which participants regard rules as valuable and as deserving of their observance. Logically, such an understanding cannot be part of the formulation of any given rule or set of rules, but is a separate feature that defines practices.

Long-term care differs strikingly from acute-oriented hospital-based care. Some long-term care, like hospital care, is residential, but the latter is usually temporary and a return to normal activities and home is typically a reasonable goal. Most long-term care, however, does not occur in institutions at all but in the elder's own home. This fact makes quite a significant difference. In the case of hospital care, the temporary nature of the hospital stay coupled with the patients' (and families') desire and belief in its therapeutic benefit underlie acceptance of the loss of autonomy that patients regularly endure in hospitals. For example, the lives of patients are regimented. Restrictions are placed on when and if routine personal care such as bathing or showering can be undertaken, when and what foods and liquids may be consumed, what visitors one might entertain, the times during which one must sleep or awaken, and there is the tacit expectation that medication be taken and other "doctor's orders" followed. Typically, these restrictions amount to a lot of things done to a patient who has surrendered independence at least for the duration of the hospital stay. These and myriad other restrictions on freedom seem to be tolerated because of the temporary nature of most hospital stays and the underlying belief that a therapeutic benefit will result. As discussed above, even the therapeutic benefit is accepted by patients on the basis of the physician's inherent authority in medical matters.

It is not clear that such assumptions make any sense or are widely accepted in long-term care, certainly not in home-based care. There appears to be a widespread belief, perhaps reflective of a deep fear, that long-term care is permanent, to be interrupted only by acute episodes of illness that require hospitalization or, finally, by death. Once commenced, the process will inexorably wind down with ever decreasing satisfaction and self-worth. The sense of independent agency or self-determination that is temporarily ceded in hospital care is thought to be lost or permanently foregone once institutional long-term care begins. This occurs even though the events that precipitate nursing home care are not necessarily parallel to acute illness. Typically, the illnesses and disabilities associated with aging that bring individuals into long-term care are chronic and usually irremediable. Since cure is out of the question, it is perversely paradoxical that medical ways of thinking prevail nonetheless because the fundamental sense of the practice of long-term care seems so different from acute medical care.

A plausible general view is that any practice should reveal its underlying beliefs and values, which justify or make sense of the rules guiding the participants in the practice in question, if only they are carefully examined. Judging from the ethnographic literature, however, the practice of long-term care, at least in nursing homes, presents a puzzling and paradoxical picture. The dominant influence of the medical model is pervasively insinuated into long-term care despite the fact that the underlying values and beliefs are widely recognized as inappropriate. A fundamental contradiction exists in this important institution of long-term care that the ethnographic work on nursing homes elaborately reveals. Fortunately, despite their cultural and social importance, nursing homes do not exhaust the full practice of long-term care.

Hospital and nursing home care occurs in places that are alien and intimidating to most patients. The situation is quite different when care occurs in an elder's home. An elder, with few exceptions, is typically on native ground. Caregivers are for the most part family members. Unlike in nursing homes (and hospitals) where the problem is not how to instill caring into health professionals, the problem is how to enable those who care for the patient to acquire the skills requisite for adequate care. Home health aides and homemakers who provide necessary personal care and homemaking services can also spend significant time with the disabled elder, but health care professionals such as nurses and physicians are only episodically involved, and certainly not on a daily basis. For the most part, the family bears the burden of caring for the disabled elder; most elders want to remain in their familiar surroundings and receive care from those they know and love (Young 1990).

In light of these patterns of long-term caregiving, it is not at all safe to assume that therapeutic relationships can or should be conceptualized along the lines of the medical model. Long-term care is in reality a diffuse set of phenomena ranging from various formal and informal in-home help services, professional home nursing care to institutional skilled nursing and medical care. Long-term care is more an extended family of practices than a single practice. Due to the dominance of the medical model in nursing homes, nursing homes seem to provide a dominant model for thinking about long-term care in general, though there is ample reason to doubt the appropriateness of this generalization, especially in light of the prevalence of in-home care. There certainly seems to be much better evidence regarding institutional long-term care than home care, a fact that can be partly explained because nursing homes are "public" social institutions, whereas care provided at home by family or friends is private and, in an important sense, invisible to social scientists. Also, the development of home care services that brings more formal elements into home care is a rather recent occurrence, though one that is already receiving attention for its impact on the autonomy of elders

(Pignatello, Taylor, and Young 1989; Young 1990; Young and Pelaez 1990). Some features of home care are uncontroversial and highly relevant to the question of autonomy in long-term care.

Home Care

More elders are cared for by their families than are found in institutions. The single largest group of caregivers are elders themselves, mostly spouses. Chronic care, in which day-to-day supervision or nursing is needed, seems to be the special province of family members. Elders seem to prefer family care over other formal and informal supports. Given all the evidence, one can conclude the norm of filial responsibility, despite its problems, enjoys significant compliance (Christiansen 1983: 27–28). Honoring these responsibilities, however, can be onerous. Even corporate America has become aware that its employees have family caregiving responsibilities that affect the workplace. Elder care has been described as an emerging employee benefit of the 1990s (Azarnoff and Scharach 1988).

For the most part, women are in the middle of the dependent care continuum; they have responsibilities for parents or sometimes for grandparents on one side and their own children on the other. No doubt this introduces significant stresses. One observer has captured the intergenerational dimension of balancing responsibilities to children with responsibilities to elder parents with the phrase "the sandwich generation" (Brody 1985). With the growth in the elderly population, it is no wonder that political programs have spurned the development of home health care from a cottage industry into a formal sector of health care beginning with the passage of Medicare and Medicaid in 1965. The number of Medicare-recognized home health care agencies increased more than 400 percent from 1966 to 1987 from 1,275 to 5,953 (Rappaport and Wood 1989). These developments have prompted reflection on the unique question of autonomy in home care settings (Dubler 1990; Kapp 1990; Pignatello, Taylor, and Young 1989; Sabatino 1990a; Young 1990).

Because home care includes various homemaking, social, as well as medical or nursing services, it hardly matches the medical model described earlier. In that model, the sick person's needs are defined in largely medical terms and managed in a professional, bureaucratic fashion. The sick person is expected to cooperate with therapy and to adapt to all its inconveniences with the goal of returning to normal functioning. Care for chronic conditions of old age rendered in the home, however, does not meet these basic conditions. Not only is cure impossible by definition, but the mode of "treatment" frequently consists of services that are in large part aimed at fulfilling the elder's daily living needs. Many are basic housekeeping or help functions, not specific nursing or medical services. In this context, there is no overriding authority comparable to that wielded by the physician in the medical model, understandably so because many elements of home care are relatively nonmedical in scope.

Informed consent that operationalizes the principle of autonomy in the acute medical care model is not of central import in the home care setting because its foil, physician authority and physician-determined beneficence, are not readily apparent either. The elder is thus in a far better position to express her own values and beliefs and to maintain independent decisionmaking. A largely ignored concern, though, is the implicit decisionmaking made by spouse and children regarding various aspects of home care. This need not be a usurpation of the dependent elder's autonomy. Even when the family makes most of the key caregiving decisions, these still could be made with the approval of the dependent elder who willingly places herself in the hands of loved ones. What seems called for is an alternative to both the individual patient rights model and the virtuous (beneficent) practitioner model, a complementary alternative that Harry R. Moody termed a "communicative ethic based on deliberation and negotiation" (1988: 69). Such a model would have to incorporate the responsibilities of the elder to reach accommodation with family caregivers (Dubler 1990). Indeed, the concern for abuse and exploitation in the home care setting, though certainly present in some cases, needs to be directed as much to caregivers as elders because the balance of power frequently favors the elder. This fact alone is reason why philosophers should pay attention to home care.

Reciprocity in the home requires that autonomy as negative freedom be augmented by more positive notions that amplify the virtues and responsibilities of elders (Jameton 1988; May 1986). Responsibilities of elders constitute a significant, yet insufficiently recognized aspect of autonomy. They comprise a part and define the limiting edge of autonomy. It is reported that patients often assume responsibilities in health care settings and that caregivers attribute responsibilities to them (Kelly and May 1982; Tagliaczzo and Mauksch 1979). If such behavior occurs to any significant degree, it prompts questions regarding its function in defining the social world of elders in long-term care. Responsibility implies a relationship with others, a relationship that is, at least implicitly, reciprocal. Responsibility relationships are not static but dynamic, changing as circumstances and capacities alter; ultimately, how one carries out one's responsibilities contributes centrally to defining the kind of person one is.

Andrew Jameton (1988) pointed out that responsibilities in long-term care are actually quite complex. These responsibilities include at least the following general kinds: first, responsibility for performing specific tasks including some of the work that is done in the institution or home, such as pushing other patients confined to wheelchairs, sewing for others, assisting in fixing beds or meals, and so forth; second, responsibilities to caregivers such as feeling a debt of gratitude expressed by gifts to caregivers, responsibility for complaining appropriately and understandingly to caregivers, and basic responsibilities not to hit, insult, or otherwise abuse caregivers that would apply to all persons generally; third, responsibilities with respect to customs and daily routines in the home of a child caregiver or institutional rules; fourth, responsibilities to other patients and residents, such as helping one's peers gain access to care, giving advice, lending assistance in activities of daily living, or showing consideration to one's family caregiver including reciprocating care and concern as much as possible; fifth, personal responsibilities regarding self-care and grooming; and sixth, responsibilities to others outside the home or institution, for instance, maintaining contacts with relatives or observing birthdays or significant life events. Even elders with limited physical abilities can assume some of these responsibilities, though, like all responsibilities, these naturally conform to changes in capacity and circumstance and in large part reflect who an elder is and what are her defining beliefs and values as a person. An elder's failure to assume these kinds of responsibilities can attest to her isolation from a sense of family or social community and a deficient sense of personal worth as a moral agent.

If frail or incapacitated elders appear powerless, they can be empowered precisely by acknowledging them as responsible persons. Taking elders seriously as members of the moral community of persons entails understanding their obligations and responsibilities as well as respecting their rights. Failure to criticize elders may subtly remove them from the realm of persons; unlike very young children who are not usually held accountable for all their actions, elders are morally mature. To respect elders as moral agents, then, requires that we acknowledge and support the virtues and character traits appropriate to being old. Virtues involve not only the habits that allow us effectively to exercise our agency in the world, but comprise the strengths that grow out of adversities and sustain us through them (May 1986: 50).

William F. May (1986) complained that academics frequently think of themselves as critics of the arrogance of caregivers, but that they, too, contribute also to the power imbalance by concentrating exclusively on the ethics of caregivers and neglecting the ethics of care receivers. Ethics cannot adequately respect or enhance the moral being of elders in long-term care if it simply clears out a zone of indeterminate liberty for them while remaining indifferent to its particular uses. A liberty merely patronized is a moral being denied. Respect for the elder as person demands more than giving him berth, licensing him to do, say, or be whatever he pleases. Respect must include an additional moral give-and-take, a sometimes painful process of mutual deliberation, judgment, and criticism, and an occasional accounting for one another's views and deeds (May 1986: 48).

Taking the autonomy of elders seriously, then, involves exploring the kinds of moral bearing that old age requires. This is equally an issue in nursing homes as in home care, but home care presents unique complications owing to the power that the elder maintains residing on her own turf and to the submerged dynamics in family relationships that invariably complicate matters. A new complication in home care is the introduction of professional caregivers of various sorts into the home bringing with them alien (to the particular home or household) models of care and routines rife with strife.

The professionalization of home health care services under Medicare has had enormous impact on the development of home care. Medicare, the only wide-based, nonmeans-tested entitlement for home care, requires that agencies providing home care be certified and licensed. Individuals are virtually precluded from qualifying as a licensed provider. Medicare takes the most severe position of all requiring that the client be homebound to qualify for home health care. Often a "case manager" is introduced and serves as an assessor who has final authority to decide what services are to be given, how often, and under what circumstances. Elders, of course, have rights of refusal, but such rights are extremely costly for frail elders to exercise. The costs associated with such a refusal are not only individual but also social. Some kinds of care cannot be refused or are more difficult to refuse because of the way it is proffered.

Some caregiving involves special social relationships. Attached to these special relationships are sets of social expectations and obligations that importantly influence and structure individual behavior. In our society caregiving relationships such as parenting, teaching, or doctoring carry rather strong normative beliefs and values that influence the kind and range of options that individuals typically envision. The injection of bureaucratic elements of the medical model into home care, even if still limited by many factors, is a cause for concern and further research. For one thing, it introduces a kind of abstract concern that if not tempered with judgment can fracture family relationships over technical issues of care when the emotional support and affective comfort provided the frail elder by spouse or children outweigh any medical benefit that specialized professional help or institutionalization could ever bring.

Until the passage of the 1987 Budget Reconciliation Act there were no specific client rights defined for home care services. By 1989 only 15 states had developed specific client rights articulated in statute or regulation. The Commission on Legal Problems of The Elderly of the American Bar Association (ABA) examined the effectiveness of these "bills of rights" to enhance or at least prevent diminution of the autonomy of elders in long-term care (Sabatino 1989; 1990b). Virtually all the rights delineated in the statutes or regulations fall into one of five categories: informational rights (e.g., to be informed regarding services available from the agency or community, charges for services, one's medical condition, name and method of contacting the provider's supervisor, and the affiliation of the agency with any organizations from whom or to whom referrals are made), participation and control rights (including participation in care planning, consent to or refusal of treatment, participation in evaluation of care, and access to one's clinical records), general civil rights and protections (to be treated with consideration, respect, and dignity, to be free from discrimination or from physical, psychological, or chemical abuse, to respect privacy and confidentiality of records and other information), remedial rights (such as to complain without fear of reprisals, to be told how to complain to the provider agency or state and local authorities), or quality rights (rights to safe and professional care, continuity of or timely care, or to be served by trained and competent personnel) (Sabatino 1990a: 22).

In reflecting on the two surveys of home care patient rights conducted by the ABA's Commission on Legal Problems of The Elderly, Charles P. Sabatino questioned whether rights language is at all appropriate to convey the positive expectations that the regulations intend. He noted that as the research proceeded, it became clear that the means of communicating with patients about their substantive legal rights, when expressed in rights language, deviated from the way elders actually thought of home care providers. Rights language sounded to most elders as adversarial and therefore posed a problem for elders who generally believed their caregivers were not even potentially their adversaries. When rights issues were reiterated in terms of *expectations* about home care, however, clients were more readily able and willing to respond. This was not simply a semantic distinction, but indicated fundamentally different ways about thinking about the nature of the relationship that the home care provider has with the elder that poses interesting questions concerning education of elders regarding their legal entitlements (Sabatino 1990a: 23–24).

These findings reinforce the point expressed earlier regarding the need for an alternative way to conceptualize respecting the disabled or frail elder in the home. The language of rights is just too strident and distracting in the intimate space of the home. Notions of filial responsibility seem far more promising as does acknowledging that to be an autonomous moral agent entails that one act with responsibility and be capable of accountability for one's decisions and actions. An ethics of home care, unlike medical ethics or an ethics of nursing home care, cannot comfortably rely on an advocacy of the elder. The elder at home is, after all, not always powerless. The ethic of strangers that patient rights supports seems singularly misplaced in the home setting. Instead, an ethic of intimates is sorely needed.

Summary

The question of autonomy in long-term care is entangled in the mythology surrounding aging and long-term care in our society. Specific treatment of autonomy in long-term care has to start with a recognition of the particular context of care and the specific care functions involved. Long-term care is a rather diffuse set of caregiving activities ranging from housekeeping help in the home to skilled nursing home care. If to be autonomous does not mean absolute independence, but involves a situated or contextual freedom, then those social institutions and relationships comprising long-term care have to be examined in some detail in order to identify practices that enhance or thwart autonomy. This would include not only how decisionmaking actually occurs, but the actual daily routines and styles of caregiving as well as the environmental features that enhance or thwart autonomy.

It is important to realize that respect for autonomy cannot mean that caregivers are absolutely precluded from influencing the decisions of elders. To be exposed to influence is not to be enslaved. In fact, we need to acknowledge that the relationship between the receiver of care and the caregiver is far more complicated, especially in long-term care, than the standard medical model implies. As discussed earlier, the paradigm assumes that the health professional is in a position of power and authority over the patient. Hence, the patient must be protected from this power and authority. In some long-term care settings, especially when care is provided by family or in the patient's home or when the elder is cognitively and decisionally competent and cared for in a nursing home by underpaid and overworked staff, the situation is likely to be reversed, that is, the elder retains power and some measure of independence. This is why the elder's responsibilities as an autonomous moral agent have to be given equal weight to any claim about the value of noninterference for the elder.

Concern for these matters prompted me to argue for an alternative framework, an alternative strategy for approaching the question of autonomy in long-term care (Agich 1990c). The next two chapters carry out this analysis in two ways. Chapter 4 deals with the more typical concern of autonomy as choice and defends a view that respecting autonomy as choice requires careful attention to the values and beliefs of the individuals involved. I argue that identification is more fundamental than free choice in understanding actual autonomy. Chapter 5 presses this analysis further by laying out a phenomenological account of some of the structural features of the world of everyday life that influence what it actually means to be an autonomous agent.

4

Actual Autonomy

A significant problem with most liberal-inspired accounts of autonomy is the inadequacy of the underlying political model, namely, state sovereignty, for understanding personal autonomy. On the political model, the person is understood on analogy with an ideal autonomous political unit that is characterized by independence from the laws and governance of other states. To be autonomous in this sense is to be sovereign within a specific political domain. Influenced by this idea, many naturally think of the autonomy of the individual as analogously involving independence from the authority of others (state, institutions, or other individuals). Autonomy is thus defined privatively as negative freedom in terms of the absence of coercion or dependence (Berlin 1969: 122; Young 1986: 3). This view of autonomy as negative freedom is an intractable problem only if it proves impossible to develop a complementary positive account. A positive account is clearly necessary to address some of the pressing problems in long-term care.

It is generally agreed that autonomy is a richly ambiguous and multitextured concept. Autonomy refers to a wide range of attributes that are generally regarded with approval. This wide range of usage suggests that it is unlikely that any essential definition can be found among these various usages (Dworkin 1988: 6). The central concepts involved in discussions of autonomy, such as consent, paternalism, or respect for persons, have such widely varying meanings partly because of their employment in different ethical theories (O'Neill 1984: 173). These different articulations of such fundamental concepts have important implications for assessing autonomy in long-term care. One helpful way to approach the theoretical morass is to employ a taxonomy of ethical theories that Onora O'Neill (1984) developed to distinguish the main alternatives: result-oriented ethics; action-oriented ethics that takes an abstract view of autonomy, cognition, and volition; and action-oriented ethics that considers the determinate cognitive and volitional capacities and incapacities of particular individuals at particular times. The phrase "respect for autonomy" has very different meanings and implications in each of these theories.

Result-Oriented Theories

Most consequentialist or result-oriented ethics do not take patient autonomy to be a fundamental constraint on medical practice. For example, utilitarian thinking regards the production of welfare or well-being as the criterion of right action. Only when respect for patient autonomy maximizes welfare is it morally required. In this view, paternalistic abridgement of autonomy is not morally wrong in itself; it is wrong only when paternalistic action fails to achieve welfare or utility maximization. This point is often overlooked because of John Stuart Mill's (1978) influential discussion of autonomy and paternalism in *On Liberty*.

Mill offered such an eloquent defense of liberty that it is sometimes overlooked by proponents of autonomy that his defense is not really an argument in favor of autonomy as a basic ethical principle. Mill actually argued that each person is the best judge of his or her own happiness and that the autonomous pursuit of one's own goals is itself a major source of happiness; therefore, happiness seldom could be maximized by actions that thwarted or disregarded another's goals. The gist of this fairly standard understanding of Mill's utilitarian defense of autonomy is that we cannot make people better off, that is, promote their happiness, if individual autonomy is restricted. This interpretation of Mill is commonplace, though not uncontroversial, because there are features of Mill's treatment of liberty that simply cannot be readily squared with this interpretation. James Bogan and Daniel Farrell (1978), for example, argued that when Mill talks of happiness as the unique intrinsically desirable end, he does not necessarily mean a subjective state attained when desires are satisfied, rather he means something much broader, namely, the composite of ends that include health, liberty, virtue, and so forth. For this reason, he can regard autonomy as desirable for its own sake, even if it does not produce the subject state for which it was originally desired. On this interpretation, then, Mill is rather close to the view that autonomy is intrinsically desirable. Nevertheless, for the sake of argument I accept O'Neill's characterization of Mill's account as an example of a result-oriented theory.

The foundation of the utilitarian complaint against paternalists is that they *miscalculate* rather than pursue welfare for another and thereby *violate autonomy*. The central place that Mill assigned to autonomy in *On Liberty* is rather anomalous in his overall result-oriented ethical theory (Dworkin 1983). The impression that autonomy is primary in this account is thus misleading because, in fact, consequences are primary for Mill and utilitarians, not free action. Apparently, because Mill believed that respecting autonomy leads to the consequences desired, namely, the maximization of welfare, autonomy—or more accurately liberty—is supported as a basic social value.

Utilitarian theory requires that one calculate expected utility or welfare based on empirical evidence and act on the results of such calculations. This is an important, yet often conveniently overlooked, feature of utilitarian thought. It is important because in empirical terms Mill's claim that respecting liberty or individual free choice will lead to a maximization of welfare or utility may be false. For example, people may be happier under beneficent policies even when these reduce the scope for autonomous action. It would be an exaggeration to say that the matter is empirically settled; it is simply not clear that individuals do prize autonomy above happiness or welfare to the degree that Mill (along with many other philosophers) assumed. Instead, many individuals seem to want relief from hard decisions and the burden of choice associated with autonomy. This also seems to be the case with much medical decisionmaking. If so, then the utilitarian defense of autonomy against paternalism fails or is seriously weakened. If this line of interpretation is correct, what follows from this conclusion?

One way to read Mill's argument is as a defense of *political* liberty or non-interference and not autonomy of persons as an ethical value. As such, it is plausible that *On Liberty* contains two distinctive, but not necessarily consistent, arguments: a utilitarian, result-oriented argument and a nonconsequentialist argument asserting that autonomy is a fundamental and irreducible condition of being a moral agent. O'Neill adopts the former interpretation. Even in this view, Mill's account is still compatible with my earlier defense of the liberal theory of *political* autonomy. As an argument regarding the public, and hence political, merit of liberty, Mill's defense of liberty is important, even if the theoretical grounds of that defense are themselves questionable or subject to exegetical dispute. For present purposes, it is sufficient to note that the enthusiasm with which antipaternalism is touted as a corollary of autonomy in medical ethics appears paradoxical, if it is true that one of the core antipaternalist texts is not itself a defense of autonomy as a fundamental value, but only as instrumental for social welfare.

Assuming that Mill's treatment of autonomy in *On Liberty* is a central example, result-oriented theories characteristically treat autonomy as a justified ethical value not in its own terms, but in terms of more fundamental considerations. The uncritical acceptance of patient autonomy and patient rights as central to medical ethics seems partly due to the function that they provide in curbing the power and pretensions of health care providers, not because they have been systematically justified in their own terms.

Action-Oriented Theories

Autonomy as an ethical concept can have a truly central place only in a different kind of ethical framework. An ethical theory that focuses on action rather than consequences is required to fully appreciate the preconditions of human agency as fundamental. Autonomy is a central presupposition of agency; therefore, action-centered ethics must take the autonomy of agents to be a basic rather than—as we find in utilitarian theory—a derivative ethical concern. This is true no matter how the fundamental ethical category is defined in any particular action-centered ethical theory. Regardless of whether human rights, human worth, personhood, or principles of obligation is the basic category or concept, autonomy is involved. This concern for autonomy is commonly expressed, following Kant, as an obligation not to use others as means, but to respect them or treat them as persons or as ends in themselves. One main implication of this view in medical ethics is that informed consent is imposed as an obligation on health professionals and that coercion or manipulation is proscribed.

O'Neill (1984: 174), however, pointed out that action-oriented theories are not equivalent or of the same kind. Some view autonomy in abstract or formal terms, for example, as a transcendental precondition for the possibility of morality (Kant), whereas others see autonomy as a concrete existential condition of being a person or moral agent. This distinction between abstract action-oriented and actual action-oriented theories is crucial for long-term care (Agich 1990c). Both kinds of action-oriented ethical theories—like result-oriented ethical theories—have to face empirical difficulties that are especially pertinent in long-term care, but abstract theories are burdened with a model that seems particularly inept. Some individuals in long-term care clearly lack cognitive and volitional capacities that would warrant thinking of them as autonomous. It is not very helpful to deal with these cases by retreating to idealized examples that avoid the fundamental question: If autonomous action is ruled out because of this lack of cognitive and volitional capacity, then what is the ground for insisting on respect or support for autonomy?

This question is central to the present study of the place of autonomy in long-term care. It is also important for medical ethics generally since patients routinely have reduced cognitive and volitional capacities. In fact, the standard view of illness is that illness represents a fundamental compromise or ontological assault on the existential conditions necessary for action in the world (Pellegrino and Thomasma 1981: 207–8). This fact, however, does not undercut the relevance of agency-centered or action-oriented ethics for medicine because many patients have *some* capacity for agency. As O'Neill (1984) argued, agent-centered moral theories can be made relevant to medical ethics if they are based on an accurate assessment of the realities of human autonomy and human personhood; she rightly pointed out that the central line of discussion in agent-centered ethics, however, has not been helpful precisely because it has tended to assume an abstract and inaccurate view of autonomy.

This abstract view of autonomy has its roots in Enlightenment political theory and particularly in the work of John Locke (1980). The consent of citizens to their government was regarded as the basis for legitimating governmental action. By consenting, citizens became the ultimate authors of governmental action. The sovereignty of the people simply means that they have consented to and so authorize the laws by which they are ruled through a contractual agreement. This contractual view assumes that individuals are autonomous, rational decision makers. As conceived in Enlightenment political theory, a theory that forms the roots of modern liberal thought, autonomy focuses on independence of action, speech, and thought. The ideals implicit in this concept include independence and self-determination, the ability to make rational and free decisions, as well as the ability to identify accurately one's desires and to assess what constitutes one's own best interest. In this view, to be a person is by definition to be capable of free and rational action. Such abilities provide the ethical foundation for expression of what are taken to be uniquely individual beliefs, desires, preferences, and values. No consideration is given to the fact that beliefs, desires, preferences, and values might be social-derived or influenced, except in circumstances in which they are imposed on unwilling individuals. Decisionmaking is regarded as a rational process that merely involves the weighing of alternatives; and communication between individuals is thought to involve primarily, if not exclusively, an exchange of information. These assumptions about the nature of persons constitute a rather large pill to swallow, which is probably why most thinkers have looked the other way when dealing with this theory.

One way to appreciate the implications of these assumptions is to consider one question involved in the debate over this political theory, namely, what constitutes consent to be governed? Does consent of individuals to a political order have to be explicit or can it be tacit? A parallel debate has occurred in medical ethics regarding whether legitimate medical intervention requires explicit consent recorded by the patient's signing consent forms or whether the patient's simply having placed herself in the care of the physician constitutes a tacit consent to whatever the doctor deems necessary provided it accords with standards of care (O'Neill 1984: 174). Indeed, those who have argued that informed consent criteria are not appropriate in medical practice sometimes explicitly reject the contractual model that underlies standard justification of informed consent. William F. May's distinction between contractual and covenant ethics in medicine is a classic statement of this debate (1975). The action-oriented ethic that derives from Enlightenment political theory assumes an idealized view of individuals as autonomous. The person is an autonomous, rational individual who functions as a discrete and isolated center of self-interested decisionmaking. Such an individual is assumed to possess what Mill (1978: 9) called "the maturity of their faculties." Other well-known idealizations of human rationality, such as "rational economic man," "consenting adults," "cosmopolitan citizens," or "rational choosers," similarly exhibit the tendency to regard persons as *ideal* rational decision makers.

A different but equally influential source for abstract approaches to autonomy is Kant's account of moral agency. According to the standard interpretation, Kant viewed the moral agent in primarily formal and abstract terms. The moral agent exercises will against desire and inclination and acts through an exercise of will that is guided by a maxim or rule in which the particular contingent facts of decisionmaking are universalized thus giving the moral law to himself. That such elements are prominent in some of Kant's ethical work is beyond doubt, but the extent and significance of this formalism is much overstated. This standard view takes moral agency to be formal and abstract. On both the Kantian as well as the Lockean treatments of moral agency, an ideal moral agent is envisaged who is defined to have full rationality and freedom to act. The problem with both approaches is that wherever cognitive or decision-making capacities are reduced, paternalism apparently must be permissible. Both opposition to and support for paternalism in medicine rely on and reflect an abstract and relatively inaccurate view of both autonomy and the process of respecting autonomy.

Curiously, this entire line of thought apparently encourages combining concern for human autonomy with (weak) paternalistic interventions. The objection to paternalism relies on the presence of distinctive cognitive and volitional capacities; their absence in frail and impaired elders thus supports a rather wide interventionist attitude. Weak paternalism thus hardly provides a middle-ground solution (Collopy 1986: 18). Having reasoned that some procedure would be consented to by an ideally autonomous elder, we may feel its imposition on an actual elder, who exhibits a compromised autonomy, is warranted. By shifting the focus from what has (actually) been consented to, to what would (ideally) be consented to, concern for actual autonomy is replaced with concern for the autonomy of hypothetical, idealized agents (O'Neill 1984: 175).

Discussions of paternalism in medicine often rely on paradigmatic four-alarm cases that shift attention from concrete, complex decisionmaking to straightforward *in principle* moral conflicts whose resolution seems to be predecided by the very facts of the case: for example, adult, competent Jehovah's Witnesses being transfused or receiving blood products against their express wishes to the contrary; a lucid and rational severe burn victim being denied release from the hospital to die from untreated infection of his burn wounds; and adult, competent patients having their lives prolonged by high technology interventions rather than being allowed to "die with dignity" (McCullough and Wear 1985: 296–97). Usually, these cases are taken to be paradigms of medical paternalism involving an interference *simpliciter* with basic expressions of freedom, whereas on closer inspection they often involve autonomy exercised to protect or assert *basic moral concerns* of the individual involved: the Jehovah's Witnesses religious belief and, in the other cases, fundamental beliefs about how one will die.

These cases are actually about respect for the individual's basic moral concerns and not simply about any choices or decisions that an individual happens to make at a particular time and in a particular circumstance; freedom from interference is understandably claimed when the issue concerns basic or fundamental beliefs and values, but this condition is not typically remembered as the point is generalized to apply to other kinds of everyday cases in which basic moral concerns are not at stake in the same way (McCullough and Wear 1985: 297). If basic beliefs and values are important elements in respecting autonomy of even seriously incapacitated individuals, then something more needs to be said about the concrete conditions of autonomy. The common tendency, however, is to set this kind of analysis aside. This tendency explains why treatment of autonomy in long-term care often focuses on discrete decisionmaking conflicts involving decisions to institutionalize patients or to institute, withhold, or withdraw high technology, usually life-sustaining care. These situations readily lend themselves to idealization and often involve patients' actual (or imputed) basic moral beliefs or values, but the range of everyday problems involving autonomy does not readily fit this pattern.

Coupled with the political/legal lineage of the standard view of autonomy, respect for freedom from interference naturally becomes a nearly absolute principle; it becomes a Nozickian "side-constraint" (Engelhardt 1982). Such a view of freedom assumes that the caregiver is a *moral* stranger to the patient and that the two share no common moral ground. If these assumptions are wrong or simply do not apply in particular cases, then freedom from interference will turn out to be a rather superficial reading of respect for autonomy. Although it is universally accepted that the autonomy of *finite* beings is at stake, the concrete complexity of finitude is constantly forgotten as more abstract perspectives are adopted instead.

The Concrete View of Persons

Autonomy involves more than explicit decisionmaking, however. Consistent with the abstract approach discussed above, choice has been the focus of most ethical analysis. Actual consent is far more complex than is generally appreciated. The practical difficulty with standard treatments of informed consent is engendered by the uncritical commitment to an abstract view of persons and the consent process. Fortunately, the legalistic understanding of consent is not the only option. One could, for example, regard informed consent as a process rather than an event (Lidz, Appelbaum, and Meisel 1988).

The problem is not so much in the idea of informed consent or its legal requirements as in the implementation of informed consent in the clinical setting. The *event* model of obtaining consent treats medical decisionmaking as a discrete act that takes place in a circumscribed period of time usually just before administration of treatment. The model emphasizes providing information to patients at that time. The law of informed consent has typically focused on the validity and adequacy of the disclosure and shied away from considering whether patients actually understand what they have been told. This model is consistent with the liberal theory of autonomy in which individuals are conceived as independent, rational decision makers. Because competence of patients is assumed, the professional obligation is reduced to providing accurate and complete information necessary to make informed decisions. Needless to say, this model assumes a rather truncated vision of the ethics of caregiving and the dynamics of clinical decisionmaking.

An alternative model views consent as a *process*. In this model informed consent is integrated into the physician-patient relationship and becomes a facet of all stages of medical decisionmaking and, indeed, interaction with patients. This model requires three conditions for its implementation. First, the role expectations of both patients and physicians need to be modified from the Parsonian model in which the patient accepts physician authority to direct treatment and is required to follow "doctor's orders" to a model that incorporates a set of expectations that treats the patient more as a responsible agent capable of participating in treatment than a passive recipient of care.

Second, before patients can successfully participate there must be a match between the illness models of patients and health professionals. For such matching to occur, health professionals must be open to the views of patients, which means they must be able to listen and learn from their patients. This is probably a less difficult task than imagined if health professionals could be trained and motivated to modify current styles of interaction. For example, Loren Pankratz and Lial Kofoed (1988) helpfully describe some of the problems and pitfalls in dealing with "geezers" and discuss ways of dealing with these individuals that promote an appreciation for their rich life histories and idiosyncratic charm. They conclude that if eccentric older men are approached with interest, understanding, and respect, then half the battle is won and the conflict that these individuals are able to introduce into the professional relationship can be avoided. For this to occur, communication must become a central feature of the consent process; not simply disclosure of information, but genuine interactional exchange will have to become the norm.

A third condition required for informed consent as process is the need to clarify the values and expectations of both patients and caregivers. Often, this seemingly obvious point provides a formidable barrier between patients and health professionals. They seem to work at cross purposes, each struggling against the other.

This view of the process model of informed consent seems particularly well-suited to long-term care, whereas the event model seems to be consistent with an acute care model. Although this view is directed primarily toward the physician-patient relationship, it offers a better paradigm for long-term care than the event model. For one thing, the model understands consent as a process that permeates the caregiving relationship. It is not confined to the disclosure of information but rather includes the definition of the problem, setting goals for treatment, selecting approaches to treatment, and defining the expected outcomes and goals. For this reason, a process model of informed consent requires a continuous dialogue between health professionals and patients. This observation is not only a practical recommendation, but implies a view of personal autonomy that acknowledges the concrete empirical features and social situatedness of persons.

Actual consent is consent to a proposed action or project *under certain descriptions*; to consent to an action does not mean that we consent to its logical implications or to its probable or actual results (O'Neill 1984: 174–75). In philosophical terms, consenting is, like other propositional attitudes, opaque. In consent we do not automatically "see through" to the implications of that to which we consent and thereby also give consent to the implications. An abstractly conceived decision maker might be able to see all the implications of a choice; no finite agent can. Often, it is argued that the patient's lack of knowledge of disease or bodily processes or diagnostic and treatment nuances prevents her from full consent; disclosure by physicians of risks, benefits, and alternatives will not bring the patient to a level of hypothetically valid consent. This is assumed to be an objection to informed consent on the grounds that the attainment of an idealized understanding is requisite, yet it is hard to see why this need be true.

Even under the best circumstances, for example, in specific contractual arrangements, appeals to consent provide only a limited justification. This limitation is recognized whenever contracts are voided because of cognitive or volitional disability or because reasonable expectations about the implications of some activity or choice failed to materialize. O'Neill argued that consent in medical contexts is thus not really anomalous; consent for medical treatment does not so much present consent theory with difficulty, but actually provides exemplary cases that highlight the *typical* limits of human autonomy in decisionmaking (1984: 175). Her view is essentially correct. It points to the fact that the limitations associated with actual human autonomy are precisely the norm, though these limitations are insufficiently reflected in accounts of respect for autonomy in actual clinical contexts. Instead, concrete expressions of human autonomy are often seen as aberrations from ideally autonomous choosing.

O'Neill's discussion of actual autonomy focused on consent and decisionmaking. For example, she insisted that whatever can be made comprehensible to and refusable by patients can be treated as subject to their consent or refusal. This understanding of autonomy requires physicians and other health care professionals to take time to establish effective communication with individuals in socially alienating environments. She said, "Without such care in imparting information and proposing treatment the 'consent' patients give to their treatment will lack the autonomous character which would show that they have not been treated paternally but rather as persons" (O'Neill 1984: 175). In long-term care, however, "treatment" permeates all daily activities because therapy potentially affects the totality of the mundane existence of individuals in long-term care. For this reason, talk about discrete "treatments" to which patients can be asked to consent, if only appropriate information is given, itself constitutes an idealization that inaccurately reflects the realities of long-term care.

O'Neill, however, did indicate that when we recognize the limited autonomy of actual patients, consent to *all* aspects and descriptions of proposed treatment is neither possible nor required. Instead, she proposed focusing on the more "fundamental" proposed policies, practices, and actions: "Respect for autonomy requires that consent be possible to *fundamental* aspects of actions and proposals, but allows that consent to trivial and ancillary aspects of action and proposals may be absent or impossible" (O'Neill 1984: 176). Unfortunately, she did not tell us how one is to identify what constitutes fundamental as opposed to peripheral policies, practices, or actions. The problem clearly is that if one makes such determination without reference to autonomy, then paternalism will be unavoidable; and, if consent is focused on specific interventions, then talk of actual or concrete autonomy beyond the mere exercise of choice becomes vacuous. It is also not intuitively clear why explicit consent is always relevant for determining what values or courses of action ethically ought to be pursued.

This point, as discussed earlier, leads some to commend communitarianism insofar as it provides a set of norms that can define what one ought to do, what one ought to consent to, independent of individual choice or action. I have dealt with that position sufficiently in Chapter 2 to establish that it is not a viable alternative. However, some components of the communitarian view, such as its insistence that human persons are fundamentally social in nature, are worth refurbishing. To do so, however, requires a theory that concretely sets human agency in its proper social nexus. Although O'Neill's discussion of actual autonomy is limited to treatment of informed consent, her discussion does point toward a more adequate account. Her view that philosophical defenses of autonomy are typically predicated on accounts of human rationality and decisionmaking that are abstract and so fail to adequately come to terms with the actual range of autonomy present in medical settings is essentially correct.

As Bart Collopy noted, "such defenses of autonomy lack the empirical savvy to convince and affect medical practitioners" (1986: 27). Collopy also correctly observed that O'Neill's proposal for a contextually sensitive ethic that would protect the patient as agent even while acknowledging the frequently imperfect nature of that agency would be highly relevant for frail elders:

An action-oriented defense of autonomy would not only have to construct a defense of autonomy in the midst of impairment as O'Neill suggests; it would also have to challenge the priority given to benefit over freedom, the defining of "benefit" primarily in medical terms, the defining of "maximal autonomy" by caregivers rather than patients, the imbalances of power within the physician-patient relationship, and the shrinkage of patient agency in the face of high-technology, high-expertise medicine. As this agenda indicates, arguing for autonomy will mean arguing against a powerful mainstream in medicine. (1986: 27)

This assessment is essentially correct both as a reading of O'Neill's approach and the general problems associated with providing a concrete action-centered theory of autonomy. Although Collopy stressed the difficulties facing this line of argument, he failed to note the advantages that such an account promises for medical ethics, such as forcing attention from dramatic, conflictual cases to more typical, day-to-day encounters in which the question of moral responsibility and style of practice of health professionals become central concerns. These would not be insignificant gains.

One main difficulty that any attempt to focus on actual autonomy must face is the rather messy incompleteness and uncertainty that actual autonomy inevitably involves when compared with ideal autonomy. One is forced to say something definite about when specific expressions of autonomy are genuine and when they are spurious or misleading. One cannot simply rely on hypothetical examples of ideally autonomous action or choice (i.e., action or choice taken as ideally rational and free), but rather one needs to identify specific concrete conditions or features that contribute to or mark an action or choice being properly seen as autonomous. The problem is that autonomy is developmentally and socially conditioned, so determinate expressions of autonomy will be unique and contextually situated thus precluding adequate formulation in abstract terms. For these reasons, a phenomenological approach is required. The goal of such an account is a general framework for understanding autonomy in the actual contexts and circumstances of long-term care. Taking actual autonomy seriously entails that ethical analysis must be contextual and irremediably particular. In point of fact, this outcome is less disturbing than it might first appear if we seriously attend to the prerequisites of autonomy itself.

Autonomy: A Developmental Perspective

A theory of autonomy predicated on a concrete understanding of the person must incorporate the developmental aspects of human personhood (Haworth 1986). The idea of human development implies an end state toward which change in personal human life is directed. Jaber F. Gubrium and David R. Buckholdt point out that physical growth provides a ready model for the development of psychosexual, cognitive, affective, and moral aspects of the person, that is, development proceeds from relative simplicity to greater complexity of structure and differentiation of function (1977: 126). Despite the many differences among theories and approaches, contemporary ideas of human development and maturation share remarkably similar views of what it means to be immature and mature. Studies of childhood development and socialization begin with what everybody already knows, namely, that there is change in human behavior that can be differentially evaluated, depending on whether it appears to be moving in the proper direction, toward greater maturity, rationality, and responsibility.

Scientists who study human growth and development assume that development is something real and factual, an objective theme open to scientific analysis. Contrasting terms such as adult/child, mature/immature, competent/incompetent, and development/retardation as well as the idea of an order of stages in the cycle of life are likewise assumed. The resulting theories of development are thus unavoidably anchored in commonsense views of human growth and change. The widespread acceptance by scientists and lay persons of the importance of certain key ideas, such as life change or maturity, have glossed over the actual dynamic social processes by which change or lack of change is defined, evaluated, and shared by people in the everyday world (Gubrium and Buckholdt 1977: 129–30).

The end state or standard of human growth and development is frequently referred to by the term *maturity*. Human development is not a pyramid built from its base in infancy. Instead, development hangs from the vertex of maturity, the point toward which progress is traced. Changes in the definition or understanding of maturity thus do not simply change the description of the highest stage, but recast the entire nature of development (Gilligan 1982: 18–19). Maturity and other key concepts deriving from the everyday, commonsense world are essentially historical and social in nature. Christie W. Kiefer argued that all developmental ideals are culture dependent: "Perhaps the best example of this is the dependency of Piagetian cognitive development, and the moral conclusions drawn from it by Kohlberg, on an aesthetics that places the generality and consistency of beliefs at a higher level than ad hoc judgement" (Kiefer 1988: 5).

Lawrence Kohlberg's theory characterized mature moral reasoning as based on a deontological appeal to universal principles or rules that are oriented toward respecting the rights of other persons. Carol Gilligan argued that Kohlberg's results are one-sided because his research is based exclusively on studies of males. Her own work with female subjects yielded a strikingly different model of moral maturity, one that consists in responsibility or the nature of certain kinds of relationships that are not predicated on individual rights. Central in the Kohlberg/ Gilligan debate is the question of the meaning of moral maturity and the concept of autonomy involved therein. For Kohlberg, autonomy and moral maturity express dominant cultural beliefs about individual freedom and autonomy as independence, whereas Gilligan calls to our attention other values and beliefs, such as responsibility and the role of judgment in the actual exercise of autonomous moral decision-making. The debate has led to interest in distinguishing a masculine and a feminist ethic (Held 1987; Lerner 1986: 26; Rest, Cooper, Coder, *et al.* 1974; Saxton 1981), though the distinction between concepts of rights and responsibilities or between an ethic of obligation and an ethic of caring or concern seems to capture a good deal of what is at stake (Benhabib 1987; Friedman 1987; Gilligan 1987; Kittay and Meyers 1987; Meyers 1987; Sher 1987). Nevertheless, the interest in actions such as childrearing and parenting are injecting valuable ideas into contemporary ethical discussion (O'Neill and Ruddick 1979). Clearly, questions about the meaning of human development and why we take it seriously are by no means merely speculative, but are components of the larger practical question about who we are (Kiefer 1988: 93).

The term *development* in our culture refers to something that is orderly, predictable, and unavoidable under usual or normal circumstances. Although development involves unspecified changes, the changes are not circular or oscillating but linear; they involve an increase rather than a decrease in qualities we assume as important or ideal for the person in question. In other words, decay is not a form of development. Without an idea of an ideal end state, however, processes are simply regarded as change, not development. Because we typically assume that time is linear and not cyclical, and that nature is mechanical and orderly, rather than idiosyncratic or personlike, we also assume a corresponding end state that manifests order and fixity. Other cultures, however, have not shared these assumptions.

In the nonliterate societies, for example, consciousness is not regarded as something amenable to development; it simply is. The idea that consciousness develops would strike people in such cultures as utterly anomalous and astounding. Individuals who fail to achieve a mature state of consciousness are thought to have been interfered with deliberately from the outside by some other consciousness or agency in a way that distorted the natural tendencies of the affected individuals (Keifer 1988: 94–95). For these reasons, Keifer (1988) argued that understanding the ideal(s) of maturity is essential, if maturation as a form of development is to be understood. Determining the final end of human development thus is essential to defining the entire trajectory of human life and existence.

Gubrium and Buckholdt (1977: 1–31) distinguish seven different kinds of conventional—conventional in the sense that they are based on popular beliefs about the reality of life change—approaches to the question of maturity. These approaches share an uncritical belief that human growth and development is not so much a concept as an extrasubjective reality or entity in the world of everyday life. With this acceptance comes the notion that the ideal of development, however it is articulated, is anchored in the world and so open to scientific investigation. One might, however, adopt another approach, what Gubrium and Buckholdt term a *social phenomenological approach*. This approach sees the employment of terms, such as competence, maturity, and mastery, as elements in and products of various kinds of social acts of interpretation that they call *negotiation*, rather than as real entities in the world. So to talk about a developmental perspective is simply to point to the fact that human persons engage in various interpretive processes or negotiations in which developmental terms actually acquire their meaning and reality and that these processes are themselves described and defined in various theories broadly called developmental. Understanding this as a process of meaning-bestowal or meaning-creation is highly relevant to our focus on actual autonomy.

Autonomy, as it concretely emerges in the practical world of everyday life as opposed to the ideal world of theory, necessarily involves processes of interpretation and negotiation. So to adopt a developmental perspective on autonomy is to ask how is autonomy established in the world of everyday life through concrete interpretive processes. If autonomy is not some ideal state central to ethical theory but otiose for practical life, it must represent a rather broad set of attributes and capabilities that all or most members of society exhibit. Included in this way of framing the concept, of course, will be normative elements that affect both self-perceptions and social perceptions of each mature individual. A dominant set of norms that are especially relevant to our discussion are independence and self-sufficiency. Underlying these norms is a naive assumption that human growth and development achieves some determinate end stage yielding a finished product, namely, an independent, competent, rational, and free decision maker, though such a view is hardly tenable. Consider, for instance, the kinds of circumstances in which maturity is an issue.

Questions of competence arise in various kinds of circumstances characterized by dispute, disagreement, or conflict. In the practice of medicine competence is not an issue when patients "consent" or passively agree to a proposed intervention, but only when they refuse to follow the doctor's recommendations. Similarly, competence is at stake in other social situations such as when one party in a divorce proceedings disputes the other's ability and right to care for the children. In many, if not most, social contexts competence is made an issue when important matters are at stake. Competence and questions of maturity, which in the context of long-term care are judged by an elder's rationality, reality-orientation, or decisional abilities, usually arise when there is disagreement over the proper care or welfare of the elder. An important subject for investigation thus concerns the concrete circumstances and ways that autonomy is ascribed or refused to elders in long-term care.

Sociality is an essential feature of human existence. Without social life and the process of socialization, the emergence of an intact individual as a biopsychosocial unity capable of thought and action would be impossible. Indeed, social life makes autonomy, however we define it, possible because without the social life world there would be no space for agency. Emphasizing social life, however, does not make discussion of autonomy derivative as familiar criticisms of communitarian approaches conclude. As pointed out in Chapter 2, one can acknowledge the social nature of human existence and expressions of autonomy without embracing metaphysical commitments about the self or communitarian commitments to tradition and community as a foundation for authority. Rather, attention to the social nature of action points us away from an abstract consideration of autonomy toward a concrete estimation of actual developmental processes.

Attention to human development forces the realization that dependence is an essential feature of human existence and that our understanding of autonomy must be reinterpreted to accommodate social arrangements such as family, friendship, and community associations that make possible autonomous human existence in the first place. Dependence is therefore problematic not in itself but in juxtaposition to an abstract ideal of autonomy as negative freedom. Viewed positively, however, autonomy involves a dialectic of independence and dependence that is best described socially as involving interdependence. Dependence consequently ceases to be a universal problem to be erased or resolved, but becomes particularized in situations and circumstances, some of which may enhance or efface autonomy.

The liberal concept of autonomy focuses on independence and self-control and prescribes noninterference as a primary value. Independence and self-control each point to different features of autonomy, namely, the individual's relationship with others and with oneself. These are common delineations of autonomy. There is, however, a dimension of personal autonomy that is more fundamental than either of these and that underlies the various social attributions of competence as a fully autonomous agent. Both independence and self-control qualify behavior, but being able simply to act is itself an achievement that is highly relevant to considerations of autonomy. As Lawrence Haworth pointed out:

> No one begins life as an agent. When for the first time the corners of an infant's mouth turn up, the infant isn't smiling. The first time the rattle falls from his hand he isn't dropping the rattle. Agency is an acquired ability. By exercising the ability, the infant builds a repertoire of performances appropriate for various needs and occasions. He learns how to get his mouth to the nipple, how to get attention, how to stand and walk. "Competence" presupposes the ability to act and refers to the adequacy of the repertoire.
> The root phenomenon is the trying (undertaking, endeavoring). . . . "Trying," in turn, is the root of "intending." (1986: 13)

Passing from barely "trying" to full-fledged "intending" consists in bringing into focus what one is trying to accomplish. Haworth argued that by barely trying the infant establishes herself as a minimal agent. The development of competence beyond this level consists in becoming able to produce intended effects. In this way, he traces the beginnings of autonomy back to the individual's first signs of *competence as an agent*. The competence at issue is admittedly minimal, indeed, nascent, but nonetheless crucial to autonomy.

Haworth argues that humans possess a basic "competence motive," a motive that involves the effort to be an agent, to gain control over one's environment, and, beyond this, to expand control by developing both a specific repertoire of skills and a generalized coping ability (1986: 55; White 1959; 1960). He points out that maintaining this minimum sense of competence is the infant's first project; the ability to do so often against odds strongly suggests that the disposition to do so is part of the equipment that the individual brings on entering the world. As a wide range of work in developmental psychology has shown, this disposition is a general or universal human potentiality (Haworth 1986: 55).

Although Haworth correctly identified effort with the "competence motive," he ties it to autonomy in a far-too general way. The competence motive and the phenomenon of trying are important not as universal conditions but because of the inescapably particular and determinate way that they are manifested in individual lives. Autonomy is not a logically necessary outcome of human development from infancy onward, but rather an empirical and altogether perilous process of achievement that occurs in dynamic interaction with others. To be autonomous is to be a particular agent individualizing oneself in particular circumstances through effortful striving in the shared social world. The striving, however, does not have an ideal of autonomy as some pregiven and logically assured end state, rather such striving *is* autonomy in an inchoate or nascent form. The striving may take many actual forms, both because individuals are not all alike and because as each individual matures competencies will be individually determined or biographically achieved; as a result, the form and substance of autonomy will be uniquely expressed in each individual's life.

For these reasons, autonomy is best not regarded as an end state of being or stage of development universally achieved once and for all, but as the precarious active engagement of particular agents in the world. To be autonomous is to be bound not only to others and history, but to the forces of contingency and luck (Nussbaum 1986). Autonomy is thus not simply a metaphysical given or an end state, but the complex process of interpretation or negotiation that is the hallmark of how individuals actually live their lives. Paradoxically, autonomy is manifested only on the basis of or in light of a background or sedimented sense of self. This self is never abstract but is a particular and determinate identity. To think of autonomy as a state or an autonomous subject as an accomplished entity is thus to adopt a foreshortened or conventional perspective. To speak *simply* of autonomy is inevitably to speak elliptically, if not misleadingly.

The autonomy of a so-called developed or mature self consists not simply in the achievement of an end state, but in the use of a particular repertoire of skills and abilities, desires and preferences that are themselves the products of past efforts and enactments in the world. All of these abilities or capacities are subject to interpretation by others in the complex dynamic that comprises the world of everyday life. To be autonomous, then, is fundamentally to strive and to experience the world in a precarious dialectic of habit and choice, necessity and reason.

Narrative Approaches

Consideration of actual autonomy requires that we think about actual agents in the world. How we think about actual autonomy is not a tangential concern. We should be careful not to rely exclusively on the language of general abilities or commitments that developmental psychology employs since such talk is inevitably abstract. A more appropriate approach to understand the development and meaning of actual autonomy involves the use of narrative and story. Awareness of the utility of this approach is reflected in the growing interest in biography, life review, life story, and reminiscence in gerontological circles (Baum 1980–81; Butler 1963; 1974; 1980–81; Johnson 1976; Kaminsky 1984; Merriam 1980; Moody 1984a; 1984b; Woodward 1986). The elder in telling her life story or stories about her past actively rearranges and reconstitutes memories as a way of establishing location and direction in the (sometimes alien) present world of experience; such an activity is an important manifestation of the actual autonomy of the elder to give meaning to her life.

Biographical construction, and indeed reconstruction since the process of telling and retelling stories about oneself involves creative adaptation, occurs on many different occasions. This simple truth seems to have escaped many in that people seem to regard the past as something that simply or objectively happened to the individual up to the present. On this typical understanding biography is assumed to be primarily, if not exclusively, a matter of discovery. In telling the story of one's life or writing someone's biography, one has to search out only what "really" happened to the individual in the past. On this view, the elder is not in a unique or privileged position with respect to the construction of her life story.

There are at least two elements involved in knowing somebody's past: the past itself and the knower. Typically or conventionally, emphasis is placed on the past itself (Gubrium and Buckholdt 1977: 158–91). The knower is simply assumed to be a passive net that gathers the true facts of the past or, at worse, as someone who distorts what *really* happened. Once it is taken for granted that an individual has a real past that occurred and is knowable, it becomes mostly a technical affair to know someone's past, personal history, or life story. On this conventional or typical view, then, biography is an objective depiction of an elder's life story. The other viewpoint, namely, that biography can be considered to be the work done by the biographer, is less commonly appreciated. Usually, people take it for granted that biography is always singular and individual. The fact that individuals can and do tell very different stories about themselves (Goffman 1963) is not readily appreciated, though these are quite common occurrences. Given the assumption that biography is single, incompatible stories are explained by reconstructing a new and true life story in terms of new facts, once the new facts are accepted as real or true. So, for example, a politician's career can be reinterpreted once his homosexuality is revealed. Thenceforward, the entire past is given a new, but now taken to be really true, rendition. As Gubrium and Buckholdt pointed out:

> Biographical work is a search for integrating accounts that lead to overall intelligibility. This process of integration requires a good deal of glossing, because the biography being considered is always the biography at hand. In someplace, at sometime, an individual's past is being considered. This limitation in space and time is meaningful to biographers in that the tacit background of specific situations defines "relevant" biography. (1977: 161)

This process is nowhere more evident in long-term care than in the way that elders lives are glossed and explained in terms of their alleged cognitive impairment or the label of Alzheimer's. Leaving aside whether these terms have any particular diagnostic validity in particular cases, the fact that an individual's life can be readily reconstituted and reduced through the foreshortening perspective of such labels raises obvious questions about the effect of biography on autonomy.

In contrast to such conventional or commonsense assumptions about biography, ones that assume it to be a matter of discovery of some real or true past, one could argue that life stories are not discovered at all, but rather are constructed through fairly elaborate interpretive processes. On this view, the past is not simply "out there," but exists only as it is constituted by the storyteller in the present. The *past* is what the biographer produces by reflecting on "facts" in such a way that they are made intelligible. Constructing a biography or telling one's life story is thus a constructive, interpretive process. It involves the conferral of meaning about oneself and the whole of the life course. Thus, when individuals tell various stories about themselves, each story represents an effort to make sense of the present in light of a constructed or invented past. One's past, in this view, is not an independent reality or truth in itself, but is a phenomenon constituted in the present to make sense of things for some storyteller or biographer.

The action of constructing a biography is, therefore, an important social action that occurs in long-term care as in other areas of social life. The importance of recordkeeping in institutional long-term care, for example, creates a medically oriented biography of the institutionalized elder's life course not only in the nursing home, but previously. *Charting* the care of elders is thus essentially an interpretive project that places the elder in an interpretive framework that largely excludes the elder's own sense of herself. Efforts to correct this dominance of the medical "biography" have turned toward life story and reminiscence as significant ways to integrate the elder as person and autonomous agent into this important social process.

One can, of course, celebrate a life story or a biography from a distance. A life story is not really the person, so it is much easier and more comfortable to handle. One danger associated with the fascination with narrative and story is that it can displace the reality of the person in long-term care. That danger, however, is counterbalanced by the positive effects of attending to the life story because the story is about a person who deserves respect. It is, of course, wrong to revel in some particular elder's life story as if it were a novel open to the hermeneutic gaze without a keen awareness of the person's needs, motives, and purposes, latent though they may be, in telling the story. For these reasons, interest in life story does not itself assure that the autonomy of elders will be respected. If attending to the stories of elders achieves respect for elders' autonomy, for example, by increasing the awareness of caregivers of the elder's unique identity, by teaching the young generally about the rich complexity of old age and elder persons, or by making specific individuals sensitive to the actual needs of particular elders, then gerontological emphasis on narrative and life story is defensible.

Stories, however, are themselves a kind of abstraction; they are artifices that gerontologists, like all academics, are prone to celebrate in place of the reality that they not only convey, but necessarily displace. The ethical significance of actual autonomy in long-term care is not to celebrate or exhibit being old and infirm from afar, but rather to suggest a framework, albeit a theoretical one, for making a practical difference in the life of elders in long-term care. The significant point about stories is that what people tell about their lives comprises one of the most important modes of access to what is important to them. Life stories indicate the things that people value most; they tell us who the person is and with what they most identify. For stories to function in this way, however, caregivers must listen and be open to this activity as an important caregiving function. Making an elder's life meaningfully available to caregivers—or, better still, making caregivers open to hearing elder's stories—is an important way to assure that a central practical concern of actual autonomy will be achieved.

Stories, however, require interpretation and the interpretive process needs to be open to the elder's own revisions. The hermeneutic of an elder's life story, or any particular story told by an elder for that matter, does not belong to specialists but to those who know the elder best. The stories are open only to those who are close enough to the elder to listen and hear. This is one practical reason justifying the use of family surrogates for decisionmaking when the elder is decisionally incompetent because they most likely know the elder best. Constructing a biography points out how our present actions, choices, and experiences, no matter how free and rational they appear, never float in a vacuum as philosophers like Sartre (1966) would have it, but reflect the particular achieved competencies and abilities that define the particular individual's self-identity, an identity that is itself in process.

Dependence in Human Development

The interesting and important problem posed by dependence is not in abstract cases in which it appears to constrain the free exercise of will abstractly regarded, but in contexts of actual choice and experience. The view that will or freedom in pursuing desires and preferences is fundamental is an understandable outcome of a model of autonomy that abstracts from concrete life. Is will and are desires and preferences the fundamental feature of autonomy? Do theoretical treatments of desire and will help us to fathom the nuanced phenomena of actual autonomy?

Humans develop through relationships with significant others such as parents. They do not simply exist in some pristine theoretical space as competent rational, free, and independent decision makers. The relationships necessary for human development are made possible not primarily by will, since it is through them that will itself emerges, but by affectivity that binds parent and child and individuals with one another in the everyday world. Such feeling for fellow humans is not a moral or character ideal, but a feature necessary to being a person in the world. Individuals instinctively reach out to others and the world because the intentional nature of consciousness involves an openness to the world. Reciprocal affective connections establish one of the conditions essential for human individuality. Such connection is essential to developing what psychoanalysts call *object relations*, namely, relations with the world and reality.

Affections determine who we are. This view has support in the accepted understanding of human growth and development. Formation of the rational will from primitive desires or preferences occurs only in relationship with others, relationships that are made possible through bonds of affection (Bowlby 1969; 1973; 1980). Affectivity and not will is primary to the process of developing autonomy. It is at least as important as desire because it provides the nurturing nexus for the fulfillment and objectification of desire. Affectivity is the means by which a rational will developmentally emerges. Consideration of human development thus necessarily brings forward the social and historical nature of human life. Actual autonomy can be assessed only in a framework that takes these factors seriously.

One main problem with mainstream treatments of the faculty of will as a fundamental expression of autonomy is the way that attention to choice and decisionmaking has effaced the wider context of conation. Desire, too, is treated as a relatively determinant phenomenon involving discrete objects amenable to cognitive expression. What these approaches omit, however, is of central concern for assessing the significance of autonomy in long-term care, especially for cognitively impaired or confused elders. Many treatments of autonomy ask the question "What does autonomy mean?" rather than the question "What is it like to be autonomous?" or "In what does autonomy actually consist?" These philosophical treatments have focused primarily on the concept or definition of autonomy, on what it means to be autonomous. In treating autonomy and long-term care, however, I am concerned primarily with the question "What is involved in respecting people's autonomy?" Focusing on this question makes autonomy conceived as negative freedom almost irrelevant and instead brings to the forefront the related questions "What does it mean to be an agent in the world? or "What does it mean to feel confused, incapacitated, or vulnerable?"

Human life and, hence, human development are essentially phenomena of interdependence. Individuals develop as human persons not simply because biological needs are fulfilled, but rather because psychosocial needs are also met. Consider the following thought experiment. By means of *in vitro* fertilization, a human embryo is created and allowed to develop extracorporeally. Also imagine the availability of an artificial womb capable of sustaining a developing embryo through the fetal development to the point of prenatal maturity. At term the infant is delivered into the world, that is, the infant's biological dependence on the artificial intrauterine environment is severed and the infant is able to exist as a separate biological entity in the world. At this point, imagine also that all the infant's biological needs are met through a series of robotic devices that feed and wash the infant. No strictly biological need is left unmet. Would such an infant develop into a normal human person? Assume that the infant reaches childhood, adolescence, and adulthood. Would such a human being be an individual, be a person, an autonomous agent in the world? Would it even be correct to say that such an entity had a world in the sense of a distinctively human world?

Research suggests that an intact human person would not emerge under such circumstances (Bowlby 1969; 1973; Harlow and Harlow 1962; Spitz 1965). Why not? Simply put, human development is not only biological, but psychosocial as well. What is missing from our example is precisely the necessary *human* psychosocial interaction. To be sure, one might imaginatively vary the case to allow the infant to view simulated faces in order to elicit the so-called social smile and permit robotic "cuddling," but such modifications only delay the inevitable. Without significant interaction with parents, actual human caregivers, the infant would not develop into a human person, even if she could survive to adulthood, though evidence suggests that early mortality would be quite high (Spitz 1965). What would be missing would be the emergence of a set of traits, skills, and abilities, such as human language and all the components of autonomous agency: a relatively unified pattern and range of feelings, rationality, and will that comprise the self-identity of the person. Dependence as a feature of human development is not simply a matter of privation or biological need, but an essential condition of what it means to be a human person as an integrated biopsychosocial entity.

Because we prize independence so much—given our cultural predilection against dependence—it is natural to view dependence of any sort as privative. This cultural attitude distorts the reality of human development as interdependent existence.

There are no telling senses in which human persons are not dependent on others. Even hermits are children of human parents; their thoughts and feelings are shaped by a cultural context that may be forsaken, but never completely eradicated without fundamentally losing one's own self. The fascination throughout the centuries with the idea of a feral child can be credited not simply to a fascination with the unusual or extraordinary, but rather with a realization that such an entity would be a living counterexample to our universal, though usually tacit, understanding of human beings as dependent in the social world.

Underlying the central dependence of human beings is the fact that human persons are embodied entities existing in the world. The human body is not only the vehicle for one's autonomous choice or will but also an impediment. The world, including other persons, also resist our efforts to act in and on it. This resistance represents not simply obstacles to be overcome, but defines the fundamental sense of dependence, namely human persons exist *in the world.* Human existence involves, what Martin Heidegger (1962) so aptly characterized as *Geworfenheit,* being thrown or thrownness. Humans are thrown into the world. We find ourselves in the world and are dependent on it. Achieving maturity or old age does not lessen this fundamental existential sense of dependence. In fact, just the opposite is true. The engaged activity that our culture takes as characteristic of middle age seems to cover over this basic dependence.

Dependence thus is an essential and ineliminable feature of human existence. It is an obvious feature of human development as human development is commonly conceptualized in terms of stages: infancy, childhood, adolescence, and adulthood. More important, humans are never finished but are essentially open to the future. For this reason, dependence is an essential feature of human beings, so the issue of elder dependence needs to be phrased not as a condition of being old and frail—since dependence as a general existential condition is hardly unique to this class—but in terms of its unique manifestation in the life of particular elders. Since the general existential conditions of being in the world are not my central theme, I can illustrate how the essential dependence of humans in the world is exemplified in frail elders in long-term care by discussing a set of conditions that bring elders into long-term care, namely, illness or disability.

Sickness as Dependence

Illness invariably involves a dissolution between one's body and self. Normally in the everyday world the self is experienced as one with one's action. The body is simply the vehicle for achieving ends in the world and is transparent to our intentions. I am not aware of my hand as I write. I am aware of my thoughts which are achieved by the pen in my hand in a complex process about which I am not usually aware. In illness a dissolution occurs in the normal relationship between the self, the body, and the world.

First, as a result of sickness one comes to depend on others to compensate for one's physical shortcomings. This dependence is expressed in the very social world of the patient. It includes needing help in performing activities of daily living or at least to substitute for those activities that the body cannot exercise on its own. Not only is the sick person dependent in the sense of needing immediate help to compensate for lost functions, but the sick person becomes dependent in a second sense in needing to rely on experts to remove or to ameliorate the first dependence. Sickness typically involves the social expectation that a professional has determined that one is legitimately in need of special care and is exempted from normal social role activities (Parsons 1958; 1975). For the elder this exemption may not involve the world of work. The "exemption" instead frequently means that the elder is deemed unable or incapable, at least without undue risk to oneself, to carry out the normal activities of everyday life including self-care activities.

The sick elder is dependent, sometimes pervasively so, on others in a way that is atypical for most normal adults. This situation leads either to experiences of hope and trust or despair and mistrust as the sick elder accommodates the dependence associated with the incapacity as well as the need to rely on caregivers for help in dealing with the first dependence (Bergsma and Thomasma 1982: 177). The dependence of the frail or incapacitated elder can cause a specific infantilization as the elder finds herself needing supervision and help with basic activities of daily living. In a variety of ways the sick elder is placed in the hands of others. Given the expectation of recovery and resumption of normal social role activities associated with being sick in our society, it is a constant source of frustration for sick elders since this usually powerful expression of hope is recognized as pallid and counterfeit. Talk of recovery or doing better can understandably be perceived as mockery or ridicule by an elder who has not adapted to this new state.

In a sense, the world is judged and experienced by the degree and kind of care that others are willing and able to extend. It also is structured by the degree and kind of care that the sick person is willing or able to accept. This latter point is important because we sometimes think that the diagnosis determines in an objective fashion the degree or kind of help that should be offered by others. As pointed out in the previous chapter, this mistake is one of the systemic problems facing long-term care. There is no objective measure of "seriousness of the illness." Illness is a subjectively experienced phenomenon. To a great extent, then, the sick elder is completely dependent on the ways that others perceive the illness. When there is a discrepancy between the perceptions, when the illness for which there is no medical cure is nonetheless viewed only in medical terms, a greater chance for despair and frustration is assured (Bergsma and Thomasma 1982: 179). The problem is less an issue of dependence as such than the meanings that dependence imposes on the particular elder.

Insofar as care is taken over by another, one becomes disengaged and alienated from the normal and everyday activities through which one relates to oneself. There is no alternative. This state of affairs is simply unavoidable. The patient thus surrenders not simply a part of her body to the caregiver, but the essential part of the self. That is probably why most elders, and people in general, prefer care rendered by those with whom they share bonds of affection, rather than strangers no matter how well trained or qualified they may be. It is indeed ironic that so much effort is expended in trying to eliminate affect from the professional caregiving or treatment relationship, when harnessing the positive affect could help avoid job and career routinization. As Julius R. Roth pointed out:

> The way to avoid job and career routinization is to put the caretaking tasks into the hands of those for whom the patient is also a special case, namely the people who love him.
>
> Let us consider the matter of caring for a sick person. There are signs to watch for, perhaps equipment to check on, medicines and other treatment to give. When such care is turned over to hired hands (as it routinely is in hospitals in our society), it is scarcely surprising that a great many errors (mostly errors of omission) are made. The patient is a victim of job routinization. He is not the special case of anyone who has his interest primarily at heart. He is dependent on people who will tend to him if they remember, if they consider it appropriate to their job, if he has not demanded 'too much' from them already, and if they do not have too much else to do. Here indeed is affective neutrality at work with scarcely inspiring results. (1973: 175)

In the tension that occurs between the self and body as a result of physical disruption, anxiety occurs. Anxiety is generally at the root of our everyday existence; a fundamental anxiety regarding death and finitude underlies all our actions in the social world. This anxiety explains our readiness to engage in the world at almost any cost. Actual autonomy for finite persons thus consists in acting in the face of death, despite the fact that all effort seems inevitably to come to nought. In the everyday world, this anxiety is channeled into individual projects and actions, and so is usually suppressed. It is brought forward, however, by illness because illness reminds the individual of the fundamental gap that exists between one's self and one's life, one's actual existence in the world.

The second consequence of the disruption in the unity of body, self, and world occasioned by illness and disability is an increased concern for the body. We usually take our bodies for granted. Even devotees of healthy living take their bodies for granted in the sense that they are not reflectively aware of bodily functions and processes as they actively pursue the goal of health. The avid jogger, for example, might be motivated by the desire for cardiovascular health and fitness or the exhilaration of exercise, but is usually unaware of the effect of running on the legs, that is, until an ankle or knee injury stops this singleminded pursuit. Illness, whether caused by specific disease processes or the normal process of aging, draws the attention of the elder to the body. Periodic or episodic attention to the body is normal, but for most adults is relatively confined given the episodic character of illness. Also, since most adults are actively engaged in the everyday world meeting the demands of work and everyday existence, pains and discomforts are regularly discounted. Illness or the feeling of something being not quite right is set aside by the active person in pursuing projects. Most adults don't have time to be sick and as a consequence may delay investigation or treatment of the illness or deny its occurrence. This behavior occurs when the individual is actively engaged in the social world; it seems adaptive in cases of most minor, acute illnesses.

In the case of chronic disease, however, individuals must acknowledge and accommodate themselves to the illness if they are to manage. In a sense, such individuals must actively work to modify their behaviors and expectations to accommodate the limitations imposed by chronic disease processes. Elders suffering with chronic disease naturally fixate on bodily processes. As a result, bodily signals such as fatigue or pain are attended to to a greater extent. The attention is not the neutral and disinterested gaze of an abstract consciousness, but is laden with concrete meanings and values. When the meanings are unclear, it is more difficult to interpret the signals. The more suspicious the interpretations, the more uncertain and anxious the patient becomes (Bergsma and Thomasma 1982: 179).

These bodily signals, however, are not meaningful in themselves but require interpretation. Uncertainty makes communication of information and participation in the process of identifying and interpreting the meaning of signals and symptoms by others important. There is good evidence that providing patients with information, for example, before surgery regarding the experiences they should expect postoperatively, is associated with better outcomes (Lindeman and van Aernham 1971). Such communication strengthens not only the patients' trust in their own bodies, but also in the caregiver who predicted and correctly interpreted the effects (Bergsma and Thomasma 1982: 179). It is often forgotten by caregivers that the attention patients give to bodily processes is necessarily part of the interpretive effort to make sense of a fractured world that is reduced to or focused on the body. The activity of interpretation is familiar, but the focus is strikingly different because the field of view, so to speak, is truncated. Hence, an increased egocentrism frequently ensues (Bergsma and Thomasma 1982: 180).

Increased egocentrism means that whenever a threat to the existence of the self is experienced, attention is immediately focused on the ego or self. In a sense, temporality is distorted and the past and future are subsumed into the present and modified by concern with illness. Egocentrism and dependence are compatible, though in necessary tension. Given this tension, it is not surprising that ambivalence is a frequent result. It is often very difficult for caregivers or even elders themselves to know whether their frustration is with the caregiver or with themselves and their situation. Hence, because of the essential connection between the sick individual and others in a caregiving relationship, they are impossible to separate completely. This symbiotic relationship, however, is not always negative, though it is always a potential source of stress because positive intimacy, too, occurs.

Intimacy in this context refers not simply to a familiarity or to a relationship structured by bonds of affection, but to a closeness or proximity of the other to the sick elder in such a degree that it is sometimes difficult for the sick elder to distinguish herself from others. It is thus hard to ascertain whether expressions of frustration or anger are directed at herself or caregivers. Frustrations also occur on the part of caregivers; it is important here that caregivers distinguish their own frustrations regarding their inadequacies in caring for compromised elders from frustrations about the elders themselves. These are not simply conceptual points, but practical problems that are inevitable in these kinds of dependent relationships. Failure to attend to the psychosocial aspects of the caregiving relationship makes it difficult to conceive how one could enhance autonomy of elders in long-term care, for it is far easier in a dependence relationship to simply take over the care of the elder without ever intending to return it to the elder. What prevents this usurpation of the elder's autonomy is a caring and respectful attitude toward the elder that manifests itself in responsibly working to help the elder maintain their identity and autonomy despite the onslaught of impairment.

These general points about dependence in states of illness help us to understand why autonomy seems so alien a concept in long-term care. Autonomy is first a problem not because frail elders have their freedom limited or taken away by powerful caregivers or impersonal institutional forces, as thinkers dominated by a primarily political model of autonomy would have it, but because the existential conditions that define the need for long-term care make the concept of autonomy as independent self-sufficiency remarkably unsuited to the purposes of concrete ethical assessment. For these purposes another, fuller concept of autonomy is needed.

Autonomy and Identification

Autonomy literally means "self-rule," that is, behavior that is spontaneous and self-initiated; such behavior is regarded as action in the sense that it manifests intentionality. Human action, in turn, can be regarded as free if the individual agent can identify with the elements from which it flows; an action (or choice) is unfree or coerced if the agent cannot identify with or dissociates from the elements that generate or prompt the action (Bergmann 1977: 37). This means that identification, the ability to reflexively recognize as one's own the constituents of an action, is logically prior to freedom; autonomy is best understood on the basis of the possession of an identity or of a self having a particular determinate nature and character. Expressions of autonomy are thus enactments of who the individual is as she is becoming. The field or stage for such playing out is the social world of everyday life.

Saying that formed identifications are the precondition for the real possibility of freedom entails a paradox. Freedom stresses the priority of the self as an individual, which is precisely what autonomy is designed to support. Given that identifications do not occur in a vacuum but are socially situated, a society can work toward establishing frameworks for the development of autonomy and the exercise of freedom, while at the same time specific institutions or social settings can exhibit patterns that thwart the expression of the self or stunt its development (Bergmann 1977: 39). The concretely, as opposed to ideally, autonomous individual is necessarily caught up in the web of contingent forces and subject to the fate of circumstance (Nussbaum 1986).

Because autonomous individuals are situated in concrete social contexts, choice is always contextual. To choose x means that y is foregone. Choosing x also means that action, sometimes effortful action, is necessary to pursue the object of choice. Choice does not automatically bring into being its object. There are thus always costs associated with any choice. The making of explicit choices or decisions, however, is not the central feature of our lives; most of our lives are spent acting in habitual, taken-for-granted ways that are not experienced as explicit decision-making. To be sure, it still makes sense to speak of choice, but the choice under discussion is more tacit than overt. As with choice, so with action.

Another important and basic sense of autonomy is freedom of action. Action is an engagement in the ambient world. It is embodied choice. Some actions and choices reflect habit. The traditional concept of autonomy as rational, free agency implies that free actions are the result of a deliberative process that yields a decision defensible on rational grounds. On this view, prior reflection and decision is necessary for an action to be judged as free. Is this a tenable view? As John Searle observed in another context:

> We ought to allow ourselves to be struck by the implications of the fact that at any point in a man's conscious life he knows without observation the answer to the question, "What are you now doing?" . . . Even in a case where a man is mistaken about what the results of his efforts are he still knows what he is *trying* to do. (1983: 90)

This intentional awareness is coextensive with action and experience; it involves an intention-in-action, an essential feature of the prereflective self-awareness that accompanies all autonomous experience. Autonomy is thus best regarded as a phenomenon of the intentional nature of consciousness. The deficiency common to most treatments of individual autonomy is that they abstract from the phenomenological complexity of actual consciousness and treat autonomy as a unidimensional phenomenon.

On standard views, everyday actions or choices that are habitual or taken-for-granted are either uninteresting or seem unfree. Such actions and choices, however, are animated by a self-awareness that is an essential feature of consciousness. From a different point of view, one could argue that such actions and choices are truly free or unfree to the extent that they are consistent with the person's self-identity. The requirement that explicit rational decisionmaking underlie all truly free action or choice is an idealization that makes sense only in light of an abstract or idealized view of the self. Actual persons could not long endure the burden of analysis and deliberation that such a view implies.

For actual, as opposed to ideal, selves, autonomy always involves developed patterns. I am more autonomous because my thoughts move *automatically* through my fingers and into my computer, not less. The skill or habit of typing enhances and extends my autonomy rather than limits it. The relationship between what is done automatically in normal human experience and autonomy unfortunately has been effaced as attention has been constricted to the phenomena associated with choice and will in most philosophical treatments. In a fuller sense, specific actions or choices can be judged to be truly free or unfree not simply because the agent did perform some particular deliberative or reflective validation, but to the extent that they are consistent with the agent's self-identity. Since individuals are never fully or completely formed, but are dynamically in the process of development, "who an individual self actually is" is always an open question for the person. Thus, the person is not a slave to the past, since present choices and actions can alter the commitments and identity of the self. Such alterations, however, are more like climatic change rather than daily changes in the weather.

In the daily course of living, the question "Who am I?" is typically suspended or set aside as a conscious matter for inquiry, but that does not mean the matter is ever really closed. The Socratic aphorism that an unexamined life is not worth living should not be taken as if philosophical reflection or psychological introspection are the only ways in which such questions are explicitly opened. Existential crises or life transitions are clearly paradigmatic ways in which questions such as "Who am I?" or "In what do I believe?" come to the fore. Sickness, too, frequently forces an examination of what is so commonly termed one's "values." In daily life, however, we are able to proceed quite nicely oblivious to our own spontaneity and freedom. The daily adjustments of intentionality as our efforts are fulfilled or frustrated in the world of actual experience constitute another ever-present way that persons autonomously act in the world. Such action is not one-sided but dynamic. It is an interaction in which the world exerts its inexorable demands and places limits on our real scope of meaningful action. Lack of explicit reflective awareness or the cognitive ability to discuss such awareness, then, cannot be taken to imply that autonomy is not present; rather, the actual rarity of fully rational, reflective deliberation regarding courses of action and outcomes should serve to remind us of the idealized status of standard models of human autonomy. The failure of much current ethical theory to take this point seriously seems an example of what Alfred North Whitehead termed *the fallacy of misplaced concreteness*, namely, the error of mistaking the abstract for the concrete (1948: 52).

Self-identity is not something that one discovers as an uncharted island in the middle of a sea, but rather is something that is made by individuals in the very course of their living. To speak meaningfully of individuals as autonomous requires that we pay attention to the kinds of things with which individuals properly identify in their lives. Saying this is to expand on the slogan "respect for persons" in a way that reflects the concrete reality of human existence. Frithjof Bergmann (1977: 48) nicely articulated the central elements of such a concrete concept of autonomy. He noted that it is only for those without a developed sense of identity that freedom has to mean "absolute independence." Since they lack a substantive sense of self, they must oppose things in order to be free. This is not the case for individuals who do not share this extreme condition. The greater the extent to which individuals do identify with something, the less is the complete isolation requisite for their being free. To put the point paradoxically: to be dependent on something does not in any way diminish one's degree of freedom as long as one truly identifies with the thing on which one is dependent. If I am in harmony with something, if in fact it is me—and that is the point of talking about identification—then I need not be protected or isolated from it in order to be autonomous. The demand that autonomy be respected takes the form of an insistence on total independence either for those who lack identity or for those things with which individuals cannot identify. In other, more typical circumstances, it is unnecessary to treat autonomy as such an extreme.

The idea that autonomy involves identification and the possession of a self-identity is quite evident in Mill's classic treatment of liberty. He, too, insisted that individuals require unique and distinctive conditions for their existence.

> If a person possesses any tolerable amount of common sense and experience, his own mode of laying out of his existence is the best, not because it is the best in itself, but because it is his own mode. Human beings are not like sheep; and

even sheep are not undistinguishably alike. A man cannot get a coat or a pair of boots to fit him unless they are either made to his measure or he has a whole warehouseful to choose from; and is it easier to fit him with a life than with a coat, or are human beings more like one another in their whole physical and spiritual conformation than in the shape of their feet? If it were only that people have diversities of taste, that is reason enough for not attempting to shape them all after one model. But different persons also require different conditions for their spiritual development; and can no more exist healthily in the same moral than all the varieties of plants can in the same physical, atmosphere and climate. The same things which are helps to one person toward the cultivation of his higher nature are hindrances to another. The same mode of life is a healthy excitement to one, keeping all his faculties of action and enjoyment in their best order, while to another it is a distracting burden which suspends or crushes all internal life. (Mill 1978: 64–65)

Not only is tolerance of diversity of choice and taste a necessary adjunct of respecting liberty, but so is acknowledging the irreducible individuality of concrete expressions of autonomy in individuals. To be autonomous thus does not require that one be able to manifest ideally rational and reflective free choice; what is required is to have a developed identity.

Another way to make this point would be to argue, following Robert B. Young (1986), that personal autonomy is a character ideal. This character ideal of autonomy is expressed in three different, but not incompatible approaches: first, autonomy taken as the ideal of character that involves making decisions and actions one's own through rational reflection (Benn 1976; Dearden 1972); second, autonomy taken as a character ideal of self-realization or self-fulfillment in which autonomy is valued as a means to achieve this end (Taylor 1979); and third, autonomy taken as a way of expressing moral integrity (Bettelheim 1960). Common to these three approaches is that autonomy is regarded as a kind of character ideal or virtue. The differences between them might be regarded as differences of emphasis and focus rather than of rival conceptions of the ideal (Young 1986: 9–10).

The Paradox of Development and Problems of Identification

It might be thought wrong or even perverse to speak of *development* in connection with long-term care when what we witness is the loss of capacity or the diminution of ability. After all, development means the progression from earlier to later stages of individual maturation, progress from the simpler to the more complex. To speak of a developmental perspective on autonomy may be relevant, but applying this view of autonomy to long-term care without major qualification surely romanticizes the harsh and unrelenting realities of long-term care. Similarly, the process of identification seems to assume abilities that only infrequently occur in long-term care. If identification cannot be founded on the individual elder's own experience, it would seem to afford a ready platform for paternalism. The problem is that identification seems to imply a rather robust self-reflective ability that few elders needing long-term care actually possess. How can autonomy be useful ethically if abilities or capacities associated with it are routinely compromised or effaced in long-term care? If autonomy is truly a primary ethical concern in long-term care, then these reservations cannot be treated lightly.

Concern about the paradox of development and identification in the context of long-term care is related to fundamental questions about the underlying theory of the person or self that the concept of autonomy implies. Typically, such accounts are concerned more with ideal expressions of autonomy, with what autonomy means, than with elucidating actual manifestations of autonomy in the world of everyday experience. Such accounts are, nonetheless, relevant to the questions raised about development and identification because they set the terms of the paradox and problems. Critically discussing these theories helps us see why the focus on identification, as the core feature of autonomy, is consistent with and mutually supported by a developmental view. This discussion also provides a firm basis for the treatment of the phenomenology of the world of everyday life that comprises the next chapter.

Many recent treatments of the self view mental phenomena, such as beliefs, compulsions, desires, judgments, wishes, and so on, as occurring on various levels. These so-called split-level theories of the self (Dworkin 1976; 1981; 1988; Frankfurt 1971; Jeffrey 1974; Neeley 1974; Young 1980a; 1980b), as well as accounts that do not use this exact terminology but still view the self in ways that involve a remarkably similar hierarchical ordering of mental phenomena (Benn 1976; Bergmann 1977; Feinberg 1980; Taylor 1976), are increasingly taken to be important for explaining the problem of autonomous choice and the conditions under which it occurs (Friedman 1986). Autonomy as negative freedom seems oblivious to a range of common cases in which a person is a slave to convention and chooses in ways that derive uncritically from the social milieu (Benn 1976: 123). These cases press toward a more robust concept of autonomy that captures the root meaning of autonomy, namely, self-rule. An autonomous person in this fuller sense not only chooses in a way that is uncoerced, but also in a way that reflects one's own goals, standards, ideals, or values. Beyond the requirement that an individual's choices be free of coercion and constraint, then, autonomy must involve some kind of reflection. The rub is that if these requirements are true in any stringent sense, then many of the conditions that engender long-term care could, by definition, prevent its satisfaction.

The fact is that there are many choices that are "free" in the sense of negative freedom, yet manifest mindless conformity to convention; such cases are paradigm examples of choices that lack what might be termed *true autonomy*. As soon as this point is accepted, however, an important qualification is needed because there are no clear limits to the extent to which the self can be thought of as biologically, psychologically, and sociologically determined. The self is determined by multiple developmental influences that combine to provide a sense of identity. If this is true, then it is unclear how a person could ever autonomously come to have values that are *uniquely* one's own (Friedman 1986: 21). One well-known view holds that if the autonomous man can not adopt his motivation *do novo*, he can still judge them after the fact. The autonomous individual is still able to step back and formulate an attitude towards the factors that influence his behavior. (Dworkin 1976:24)

On this view, motivation becomes a person's own motivation so long as the person judges that she wants to be motivated as she is and so long as the judgment results from a process of critical reflection, reflection that is free of manipulation, deception, or other constraints on the process of reflection. In simplest terms, a person who approves of motivations in this way "identifies" with them. This view has widespread support (Dworkin 1976: 25; Feinberg 1980: 8; Frankfurt 1971:13; Young 1980a: 37). The process involved is essentially one of self-reflection that judges one's first-order preferences according to a second higher level of preferences, indeed, on the basis of the highest principles available.

The problem with this account, as Marilyn Friedman rightly pointed out, is the special status that it accords critical reflection. Without critical reflection, there can be no true autonomy. This poses an important problem because if such a capacity is essential, then autonomy might prove to be rather rare, especially in long-term care. Critical reflection can confer autonomy in at least two different senses: first, the critically reflective self has a special ontological role in constituting the self as the "true self." Second, the process of critical reflection may involve the agent's identifying with her motivation. Such identification is sometimes taken to have ontological significance in that critical reflection is thought to be autonomy-conferring just because it constitutes the "higher," "real," or "true" self (Dworkin 1976: 24; Feinberg 1980: 19–20). Here the liberal worry, discussed in Chapter 2, about covert metaphysical commitments in theories of positive autonomy seems to recur.

This problem is partly an artifact of the use of adjectives such as higher, real, or true in connection with the self. This language seems to imply that there is an ontologically distinctive entity or component of self that comprises its essence. There is, however, no compelling reason to think that this need be the case, even though the talk of higher, real, or true selves is quite prominent in philosophical treatments of autonomy. In connection with specific cases or examples, such talk is usually understandable and not problematic. It seems natural and unobjectionable, for example, to speak about a true or higher self if the example involves a committed parent explaining why his family takes precedence over dedication to a favorite sport. Not traveling out of town to see a team play in deference to attending a child's school performance seems comfortably expressed as an action and decision expressive of who the parent truly is or the higher values that the parent chooses to support *as a parent*.

Similarly, discussing one's religious convictions that were arrived at after a long soul-searching examination and reflection on one's previous taken-for-granted beliefs and values makes eminently good sense when expressed in terms of a notion of a higher or real self. To speak generally, especially in the context of philosophical analysis, of judging or evaluating one's first-order desires or preferences through a process of critical reflection in terms of a hierarchical apportionment of the self, however, is misleading given the tendency to reify the abstraction. The important point is that, although this mode of speaking is understandable and defensible *in particular everyday contexts*, problems occur when these terms are reified as abstract elements or component parts of the self. When philosophers speak abstractly and universally about lower and higher levels, first-order and second-order motivations, and so on, no particular point of reference exists because the terminology is frequently detached from actual agency and actual autonomy. Although I have eschewed such approaches to autonomy, it makes sense to see whether identification, that is commonly expressed in just these kinds of abstract terms, can nonetheless be refurbished with the accoutrements of actual autonomy.

If autonomy primarily consists in identification as understood by most split-level theorists, then can one adequately address the central theoretical problems that identification involves. Actions or choices are seen as autonomous only if the individual is capable of identifying with them in the sense that they cohere with the *true* sense of self. The source of autonomy, namely, the alleged true or higher self, however, is not itself necessarily autonomous to begin with. It is not clear that the *true* self is something in respect to which autonomy is already effective. In other words, the fact that a person identifies an element of herself as "true" or "identifies" with it, such identification does not itself assure that this part is truly her true self or is itself the basis of her identity. The relationship here is clearly contingent, not logical. The fact that the relationship is not logical or ontological is a problem for split-level theories. In part, the problem is traceable to the rather abstract view of autonomy and agency that characterizes these treatments. Although the problem is difficult, it is not necessarily intractable, especially in an account that adheres to *actual* autonomy.

The theoretical problem that split-level theorists must face is that critical reflection on the one hand seems to be autonomy-conferring, yet the highest principles that guide the reflective evaluation of lower-level choices and motivations, too, must be autonomy-conferring (Friedman 1986: 29). Split-level accounts typically provide no adequate explanation of the way that autonomy could be conferred by a process whose highest principles themselves are not autonomously the agent's "own." The split-level account of autonomy makes no provision for the realization of autonomy in respect to a person's highest values or principles. Nevertheless, this problem could be avoided if critical reflection did not have to be conceived as a "top-down" affair. If it must be top-down, then there is no room for autonomy at the top and that is clearly paradoxical. The way out of this morass is to develop an account in which autonomy is conceived as a two-way process of integration involving a person's higher motivations, intermediate standards and values, and highest principles (Friedman 1986: 32).

One can usefully draw on an analogy with scientific explanation. Autonomy involves the process by which a person's "covering" principles, especially those at the "highest level" are "inducted" from what *they* are suppose to cover, namely, lower-level choices or motivations. In other words, one builds up from experience, from one's actual choices and motivations, a sense of self that includes or is amenable to expression in terms of higher-level principles. This sense of self then serves as a normative principle for identification of subsequent experiences, choices, and so forth. Because this sense of self is a product of developmental influence, it is mainly an empirical product; it is not an ontological postulate. In other words, a person's higher values and principles, whatever ontological status they might have, empirically have to be subjected to assessment in terms of actual experience.

Although split-level theorists say that the higher or highest values and principles must be *able* to be judged rational by some special act or kind of critical reflection, they need not be *actually* reflected on; rather, the essential requirement is that they be *lived* and *experienced* as one's own, as cohering with the sense of one's developed self. How that might occur is an important psychological and phenomenological question, but it is not a matter to be settled by ethical theory. One relevant suggestion is that the concept of a life story and the narrative nature of life is far more important than usually appreciated by philosophers. It may well be that the coherence at stake is not ontological or logical at all, but aesthetic. If so, then standard conceptual commitments and styles of ethical analysis would need to be rather fundamentally rethought.

For a "self-concept" to become a person's "own" self-concept, then, it must have been assessed by oneself for its fitness with whatever else already motivates and guides one. It must be a product of one's own developmental history. For this reason, attention to autonomy in long-term care necessarily involves attention to actual as opposed to ideal autonomy and to the phenomenology of the everyday life of elders. This focus necessarily constitutes a "bottom-up" form of assessment (Friedman 1986: 32). In this way, then, the problem of talking about development in the context of long-term care is rendered less "perverse" than it might first appear for elders in long-term care.

Identification is a process that occurs in the everyday experience of persons; one's sense of self is both formed and confirmed in the course of this experience in the world. As noted earlier, maturity is not an end-stage of a linear process of development, but rather a particular *kind* of development, one that involves self-mastery, effective competence in the world, as well as identification. To be an autonomous person in the world is to develop, develop not toward some abstract ideal that once-attained is then forever enacted, but as an integrative process of accommodating oneself to new circumstances and adapting those circumstances to one's unique structures of meaning. Identification thus precedes autonomy as independence (Bergmann 1977).

Even relatively abstract accounts like split-level accounts can be made to accommodate the concerns expressed earlier. As a matter of fact, the split-level approach encounters its unique set of problems mainly because it relies on a hierarchical, abstract model of the self rather than on an integrated vision of the concrete person in the world. In a sense, the problems posed by development and identification are at least partly due to the metaphor underlying the discussion of choice, namely, to adapt Frost's phrase, two paths diverging in a wood. This metaphor obscures what is central in human action and choice, namely, uncertainty and the full range of background considerations that structure the perception of choices as open or viable. The path metaphor makes choice appear to be a matter of explicit options or alternatives, whereas this hardly captures the range of circumstances that are ethically important, particularly in long-term care.

Another metaphor might be more appropriate, namely, the metaphor of crossing a field of tall grass. Depending on where one entered the field or one's interests, purposes, or needs, one might follow the natural gradient, as in a leisurely stroll, or let it work against one, as an avid runner might do to build stamina. Certainly, the field might be crisscrossed with paths from previous travelers, but they will only be evident in the irregularities in the growing patterns of the grass, its deviation from the perpendicular, but not as a smooth way. The influences of others and society will be simply patterns or tendencies, not causally determining forces. One might, of course, note these ways in advance and choose the one that afforded the least resistance, but the metaphor does not require that action and choice be so constrained. There is considerably more room for autonomy creatively and individually to make its own way across the field of life. A person's action might be guided by the evident patterns marked out in the field, but they might be guided as well by literally loftier objectives, because one followed the flight of a grouse without regard for the field itself or simply ambled in a general direction or toward a specific endpoint, such as a particular tree at the end of the field.

The metaphor of the field of grass instead of the path metaphor is far more adequate for the purposes of understanding autonomy in long-term care. It is also far more apt for understanding actual autonomy, but discussion of that point is beyond the limited objectives of this work. Its chief advantage is the way it directs our attention to a wider range of phenomena not normally thought of as relevant to the question of autonomous action and choice. In the next chapter, I show that because actual autonomy involves being an agent in the everyday world, attention to certain structural features of that world can helpfully illuminate aspects of long-term care that might not normally be seen as features of autonomy.

Implications for Long-Term Care

The foregoing discussion raises at least two important questions regarding long-term care. First, are the choices actually afforded individuals in long-term care the kind of choices that are meaningful or worth making? In other words, even when individuals are afforded choices, autonomy may not be significantly enhanced because the choices available may not be meaningful for the individuals involved. Ideally, choice that enhances autonomy is choice that is meaningful for individuals and allows them to express and develop their own individuality. If such is not the case, then the true sense of autonomy of persons is not enhanced.

Consider, for example, the kinds of choices that are typically afforded individuals in nursing homes. There are choices regarding limited outings, the use of special services such as hair dressing or participation in structured social and recreational activities such as bingo. No matter how extensive this list of choices is, one can ask whether the choices are meaningful for the individuals. That is, does the list include choices that preserve and enhance their individuality and identity such as choosing when and what to eat, or "permission" to choose to ask or not ask for help from staff. If it is the case that the actual choices afforded to individuals in nursing homes are not seen by those individuals as meaningful, but that other "choices" not made available are seen as meaningful, then serious questions arise regarding how autonomy is being respected in these circumstances. This suggests that caregivers and managers must attend more thoroughly to the question of the meaningfulness of the choices actually afforded elders under their care.

Being able to identify with one's choices is a prerequisite for true autonomy. There are choices which individuals can be forced to make that negate the integrity and self-worth of the person. In the movie *Sophie's Choice* a Jewish woman was made to choose either her son or daughter for extermination on entry into a Nazi concentration camp. Although she did "choose," her choice was not one with which she could rationally or sanely identify. Hence that choice haunts her throughout life. It is a surd element that distorts her ability to love and function as a mature person. Similar, though less dramatic, kinds of choices are also confronted by elders or families with disabled elders requiring long-term care.

The seventy-five-year-old woman whose own health is deteriorating must make choices regarding the care of her seventy-eight-year-old husband who has suffered a stroke and is now bedridden. Similarly, the husband must choose institutionalization or watch as his own care consumes his wife. The family of such a couple, too, must struggle with choices that are equally difficult. Do they take the couple into their households for care? Do they break up the couple and arrange for different care for each of their parents? Are there alternatives available in long-term care that offer choices with which individuals can identify? Sometimes, the cost to self for the elder in agreeing to move in with children is too great not because the elder fears dependence and instead prizes independence, but because the elder cannot identify with a choice that imposes burdens on children and means the loss of friends and familiar surroundings.

The psychological consequence of this point is evident everywhere in long-term care. As Bergmann has pointed out, nonidentification characteristically carries with it a sense of passivity: "Once the subject structures his experience in a certain way, he *has* to feel passive, but the sense of passivity in turn reinforces the nonidentification: the self that is overwhelmed at every moment withdraws still further" (1977: 48). Thus, the phenomena of withdrawal and generalized depression that one often sees in institutionalized elders may be traced to the existentially tragic choices the elder is forced to make or live with. Recognizing this point is clinically helpful even if the situation of tragic choice generally defies solution by society.

If altering identifications is sometimes too formidable a problem or requires too long term a solution, then we should look elsewhere to address the sequelae of tragic choice. That is, if we are serious about enhancing the autonomy of elders in long-term care, but are unable to modify social and institutional patterns of care, then we must turn specifically to the ways that long-term care is locally implemented and introduce modifications that hold the promise of at least remedially addressing the issue of respect for persons. This is, in effect, the second question that autonomy as identification poses for long-term care.

If the actual exercise of choice is typically only a small part of our lives, then questions about the style of life and the structure and organization of long-term care become important. In other words, is this "style" of life available in long-term care meaningful for the elder? Is the life available in long-term care something with which the elder can identify, that is, not through explicit choice but passively and reflexively? Raising this question suggests that a radically different metaphor of autonomy in long-term care is required. In this new picture there are no walls and everything is open. There are not, as in the traditional view, decision-making nodes along a narrow path that diverges at certain points: the decision to institutionalize or to accept skilled-level care. Instead, autonomy is always present, though sometimes hidden from view as individuals go about their daily lives. Every step and every move we make could have been different, though it seldom seems to be.

We are carried forward in our lives by a constant and monotonous exercise of choice of which we are all but oblivious. Choice does not hover only between two alternatives; there is rarely just a simple fork, a stark either/or; rather, at every step, we could have moved in countless possible directions whether we realize it or not (Bergmann 1977: 77). That is why I insisted earlier that the proper understanding of autonomy involves appreciating how individuals are interconnected; how individuals are determined by historical and social factors. Human growth and development is not simply a stage through which we pass to become adult, independent decision makers, but development as dynamic adaptation and encounter with the world persists throughout our lives. Autonomy is an essential spontaneity that defines human personhood and is ever present; for example, in the acquisition of habits of action and thought, they are as much socially derived as they are individually and uniquely determined. Thus, we need to pay more attention to the psychosocial correlates of autonomy and to the arrangements which either foster or thwart the development and expression of individuality and personhood.

Taking identification seriously means facing a particularly problematic question. As discussed in Chapter 3, nursing homes are remarkably heterogeneous and complex social and cultural systems. Hence, they are fraught with potential conflicts. It is simply not reasonable to expect that ethnic or racial stereotypes that developed over a lifetime will disappear as one enters a nursing home as a resident or staff member (Foldes 1990: 24). These markers of identity do not magically fade away when people become old and sick, so the question arises what if the central values and beliefs of elders are discriminatory, mean, or selfish.

The requirements of autonomy as independence certainly support individuals manifesting and maintaining attitudes and beliefs that are not ethically defensible, but only so long as those attitudes and beliefs do not infringe on the rights of others. Concern and respect for others is ethically required. Liberal principles do not exclude this positive assertion, but also do not help much in understanding the positive ethical demands that autonomy places on an agent. It is inadequate to acknowledge that someone is truly a bigot and let matters rest there. Actual autonomy does have implications regarding how one might deal with a bigot by sanctioning appeal to the primary sense of responsibility that essentially characterizes what it means to be an agent. The account developed in this chapter indicates that actual identifications supporting true autonomy are developmentally and socially determined. Hence, concern and respect for others is not optional for the truly autonomous self, but a basic obligation because they support the very conditions necessary for a formed self. Understanding how the elder developed these views provides important opportunities for personal growth even at a time that the person's life is winding down. In a sense, one cannot speak of development in the context of long-term care without seriously acknowledging that changed attitudes and beliefs are always possible, but constrained, as they inevitably are in the practical world of life, by chance and history.

Despite the complex historical, institutional, and social character of our understandings of disease and health (Agich 1983a; Caplan *et al.* 1981; Twaddle 1979), it is clear that there is a striking divergence between contemporary concepts of health care based on acute-oriented concepts of disease and chronic-oriented concepts. In their analysis of unpublished data from the Health Interview Survey and the National Nursing Home Study, L. H. Butler and P. W. Newacheck found that almost of all of the decline in health associated with increasing age is accounted for by chronic rather than acute conditions (1981). Similarly, as L. Cluff has noted with regard to chronic disease, acute or episodic care alone is inadequate; the expectation and goal of care is and should not be the elimination of disease, which by definition in chronic conditions is not possible, but rather *maintenance of function* (1981).

Given that elders seem more likely than younger persons to experience functional disabilities as the result of chronic illnesses (Fredman and Haynes 1985), are services available that adequately meet these needs? By "functional disability" I mean the degree to which an illness or impairment interferes with meaninfgul daily living. These are often measured in empirical studies by the number of days lost from housework, school, work, or days spent in bed (Butler and Newacheck 1981). The concept of functional ability measures the impact of an illness or impairment on the individual and on the individual's ability to engage and interact in the social world, rather than focusing on the presence or absence of disease. Indeed, some have noted that "the loss or impairment of the ability to perform such basic daily functions as shopping or bathing strikes at what the elderly value most— independent living" (Pegels 1981: 5). "Independent living" here does not necessarily mean autonomy conceived as independence, but rather is consistent with the concept of autonomy as identification; it means the kind of life that coheres with the elder's own sense of self and actual abilities. The ability to perform normal functions of daily living are best understood in terms of the individual's own sense of self-worth, how the elder identifies herself, than as a desire for independence and noninterference. One challenge for institutional long-term care is to develop supportive substitutes for the activities that elders value, but can no longer perform.

That loss of function is an important concern is supported by the literature that notes a lack of association in the minds of elders between health and the presence of chronic illness or disability (Ferraro 1980; Fillenbaum 1979). In some studies, 68 percent of noninstitutionalized elders report their health as excellent or good despite the fact that 85 percent have at least one chronic illness and 47 percent have some functional disability (Filner and Williams 1979; Kovar 1977). These findings suggest that individuals experience themselves as healthy if they maintain functional ability even in the face of chronic disease. The account of autonomy just offered helps to explain theoretically why this is so. Maintaining a sense of autonomous well-being is consistent with dependencies on medication or professional care *if* those dependencies help to maintain a sense of functional integrity in those areas of life that individuals value. Dependencies do not conflict with autonomy if individuals can still maintain a sufficiently adequate range of identifications to sustain their own sense of integrity and worth.

These observations help to explain why focusing on disease and acute, episodic interventions has such dramatic implications for the concept of autonomy in long-term care. Given a disease-driven model of health care, specific decisions such as those regarding institutionalization, increasing levels of skilled nursing care, withholding or withdrawing technological life supports naturally become prominent. Correlatively, worries about infringement of individuals' fundamental rights naturally arise and so support the belief that autonomy is properly and exclusively to be conceived on the basis of independence and noninterference. In such a view, what seems less pressing and even insignificant are the mundane aspects of long-term care. Attention to everyday ethics (Kane and Caplan 1990), however, is a necessary component of any serious and sustained treatment of actual autonomy in long-term care.

Robert Kastenbaum has argued that

> we often see the clinical ambience minus the clinical benefits. The person who is a patient only temporarily can adjust to the unfamiliar and unlovely hospital routines knowing that this is only an interlude. Some comfort and individuality is sacrificed; however, in fair return the person receives state-of-the-art medical and nursing care. By contrast, the geriatric milieu is a long-term or permanent arrangement for many people, and the clinical ambience is not counterbalanced by superb care. Perhaps the most infuriating note from the standpoint of the patient is the attitude that "this is all for your own good." It is not—and everybody knows it. (1983: 11)

Although nursing dominates the nursing home, registered nurses are seldom regularly seen by residents. Licensed practical nurses (LPNs) and certified nursing assistants (CNAs) provide most care. A bitter irony for most institutionalized elders is that the disruptive move to the nursing home is predicated on their unique medical needs requiring around-the-clock care when they typically seldom have contact with a physician or nurse after their admission (Kane 1990: 12).

Kastenbaum argues that the necessary goal for the clinical milieu is less a matter of specific interventions than "making the world right again" (1983: 12–15). Frail and impaired older persons experience many sorrows, losses, fears, and frustrations in addition to the physical ailments and disabilities. A truly therapeutic environment would certainly provide treatments that ameliorate discomfort and help individuals maintain a level of integrated functioning, but would also attend to the everyday routine and quality of experience for the residents. The safest generalization one can make for the experience of the nursing home is "boring" (Kane 1990: 17). There are long stretches in which elders have nothing to look forward to except the next meal. No wonder, then, that institutionalized elders have been found to engage in activities that observers might take to be relatively bizarre and apparently meaningless such as watching cars (Gubrium 1975: 180–84). This behavior is far from passive, since it represents an engaged and autonomous activity of elders with serious functional limitations. It is an example of an elder engaging in the social world of everyday life that is quite restricted by physical and environmental factors. As Timothy Diamond reported on his own participant observation:

> I came to change my image of nursing home life as a static enterprise. It is not sitting in a chair 'doing nothing.' Rather than being passive, it is always a process. Each person is situated in a somewhat overall turbulent path. Each person sits in a chair or lies in a bed, often appearing motionless, but is moving and being moved, however silently, through the society. (1986: 1289)

Talking, walking, and watching were actually quite important activities for elders at Murray Manor. They represented various ways that elders tried to avoid "just sitting around" as opposed to "sitting around" in which the elder is engaged in some personally meaningful activity. When observed to be "just sitting," nervousness and anxiety was reported by both elders and staff; it was associated with unnecessary toileting that produced no urine or stool or other requests for staff help. The psychological and social dynamic of these requests raises the question "What are some of the relevant conditions of actual autonomy in long-term care?"

The consequence of these points is that geriatric ethics must attend to what Hans Selye termed "the syndrome of just being sick" (1956: 79), namely, that things are just "not right." Besides specific disabilities and pains, there is a sense of the world gone awry, a pervasive sense of loss or what might simply be termed "existential despair." Kastenbaum argues that the "just being sick" syndrome can be countered effectively by a milieu that accentuates the positive, namely, a milieu that develops a systematic and encompassing framework of positive expectations on the part of everyone involved. Clarifying the components of such a milieu would be one way to manifest concern for autonomy. To do that, however, requires that the concept of autonomy be refurbished along the lines developed in this work.

Summary

I have discussed result-oriented and action or agent-oriented ethical theories and argued that the latter afford a more adequate basis for conceptualizing autonomy. Unfortunately, insofar as they rely on an abstract rather than a concrete view of human persons, even action or agent-oriented theories do not carry us far enough. Reliance on abstract views of action and choice is problematic because it reduces the complex reality of individuals in health care to the idealization of a competent, rational free agent. In point of fact, such idealizations seldom obtain. Between ideal competence and actual incompetence exists a wide variation that needs to be addressed.

Core to my account of actual autonomy is the view that identification precedes autonomy and, indeed, is a more primary phenomenon in terms of which autonomy as choice would be best analyzed. Identification is a common-enough theme in recent philosophical treatments of autonomy. I have tried to show how adhering to actual autonomy solves certain theoretical problems associated with typical split-level approaches. The main point is that what autonomy actually means in the everyday world of long-term care is likely to exceed by a rather long margin the usual range of philosophical discussion and analysis that relies too heavily on rather abstract cases and problems.

Respecting the autonomy of persons in long-term care entails a commitment to identifying and establishing conditions that encourage individuals to face adversity and threats to self that are the inevitable result of the illnesses and functional deteriorations that bring elders to long-term care in the first place. Respecting autonomy requires attending to those things that are truly and significantly meaningful and important for elders. This means that elders must be treated as individuals, as unique persons with identifiable personal histories and a rich store of experiences and memories. When such identifications are difficult to assess, as in cases of severe memory deficits associated with Alzheimer's disease or other cognitive impairments, patients frequently respond, albeit minimally and in deficient ways, to direct contact with caregivers and others. Long-term care can provide positive messages and hope even in the face of serious impairment. Hope does not mean recovery, however, as is usually assumed in the medical context; instead, hope refers to the prospect of meaningful experience with others at those times when one most needs comfort and companionship. The natural tendency of long-term care to distort self-perception and the social functioning of elders must be acknowledged. The phenomenological framework for understanding autonomy that I develop in the next chapter provides some concrete benchmarks for assessing the ethics of specific long-term care settings.

5

A Phenomenological View
of Social Action

In this chapter I discuss some general and some specific features of the social world as a way to develop further the view of actual autonomy that shows the essential connectedness that binds humans together. Once we appreciate the interdependent character of being an autonomous agent in the world, the implications of autonomy for long-term care can be discussed without being restricted to the ideals of independence and noninterference. This chapter develops some general features of the social world and what it means to be a person existing in that world. Autonomy is seen as a core defining feature of persons in this view, but persons so defined are seen to be essentially connected with, rather than isolated from, others and the world. Four exemplary aspects of the phenomenology of the social existence of persons are presented: the spatial, temporal, communicative, and affective. Implications for long-term care are drawn for each of these dimensions of human existence. This discussion thus provides a basic framework for reassessing and reconceptualizing the problems associated with autonomy of elders in long-term care.

Sociality

I have discussed the liberal concept of autonomy and sketched a set of considerations supporting a view of actual autonomy involving development of identifications. The thrust of this analysis is that persons are interdependent; as agents they exist in the social world of everyday life and their autonomy emerges and has its terminus therein. These considerations can be taken in either of two directions, one well-recognized and another, to use Frost's phrase, a "less travelled path." The first is to see sociality as a guide to a communitarian ethic, an ethic that stresses human relationships, commitment, and tradition as central values. Autonomy as an ideal of the isolated, abstract decision maker obviously has no place in such a scheme. As a general theory of human nature that denies the importance of shared commitments, the liberal view of autonomy is surely suspect, but as a political

114

doctrine according to which the government should treat persons as individuals, that is, apart from status and ascription, the liberal theory is worth saving.

Distinguishing between the liberal view of autonomy as a theory of human nature and a theory of politics is crucial. Admittedly, the critics of liberalism are correct in pointing out its deficiencies as an ethical theory, but that does not invalidate its importance when brought within the compass of politics and the public life. One can preserve the essential contribution of liberal thought to modern culture and society, namely, affording a justification for protecting individuals from the intrusive power of the state and other individuals with a shell of legal rights, while at the same time acknowledging that this view presents at best a truncated understanding of the nature of autonomy, moral obligation, and the scope of ethics. Critics of liberalism, however, point out that when autonomy is taken in its libertarian form, any meaningful sense of community or tradition, which is seen to underlie morality, is inevitably lost insofar as *anything* that a free individual desires or prefers and can freely choose becomes *morally* acceptable. Such a view is ultimately incoherent and indefensible. That it has any credibility whatever attests to the degree to which the legal understanding of rights and the political understanding of autonomy infuse contemporary thought.

Communitarians, unfortunately, propose to address these problems globally by substituting a focus on community and tradition for the liberal ideal of autonomous free choice. Such a substitution, however, rejects the core tenet of liberalism, namely, that autonomy is central in a philosophy of politics, and proposes instead a philosophical anthropology in which community is central. In part, the problem with this approach not only involves denaturing the moral into the political, but attempts to resolve political and moral problems by appealing to a substantive philosophical anthropology or metaphysics. That is why it is important to consider the second approach to sociality.

On this second view, sociality is an essential feature of being human. This is a descriptive, phenomenological claim and not a metaphysical or explanatory claim as offered by the communitarian. That is to say, no normative ethical claims are made with respect to sociality as a feature of personal autonomy, but rather a set of observations is offered that suggest implications for framing the ethical analysis of long-term care.

The world of human life is inexorably a shared world. Individuals come to have a place in the world, a world which exists before birth and which is experienced as a world organized by predecessors. To be in the world means, of course, to be located at a specific place and time. Spatially and temporally I am "here" and "now"; my body is the axis of a set of coordinates which locates the world and all that it contains. In terms of this spatiotemporal location, all else is arrayed before or after me.

As individuals each of us has a different "here." This is not simply a physical location in the world, but also points to a unique biographical situation. In other words, as individuals we are biographically determined by and through those attachments and interactions with others in which we develop competencies to deal with the world. Such competencies might be termed the "stock of knowledge at hand" that is composed of the habits and skills acquired through previous experience. The stock of knowledge at hand is composed primarily of language, the multiple typifications that are employed and embodied in language, and various recipes for action, such as rules for handling and manipulating things, that are appropriate in typical situations. Much of this stock of knowledge at hand is socially derived and determined. In this sense, then, many actions and choices are prefigured in the shared social orientation to the world. The social reality around us makes certain choices appear *as choices* for us. This deterministic dimension, however, coexists with the biographically determined situation in which a unique system of "relevance" evolves. The unique orientation of each individual brings with it a selection of elements, either by affection, belief, choice, desire, feeling, preference, or tendency, that on the basis of past strivings and experience define the unique identity of the person. For present purposes this discussion of sociality is limited to elaborating structural conditions that undergird autonomous action in the everyday world and that determine elders' experience of the world of long-term care.

The Everyday World

The commonsense or everyday world provides the setting for judging the adequacy of any ethics. It does so because the everyday world is a practical world of doing, the *paramount reality* (Schutz 1971a: 226–29, 341–44), within which our lives are lived and which provides the "reality" or content that ethical reflection seeks to clarify. This world is a historical world in which human beings come into existence and acquire their standing as agents or persons. It is the place wherein their lives are lived, actions undertaken, and choices made. It is important to emphasize that the term *world of everyday life* refers to a zone of experience that is not limited, as the term might be mistaken to imply the ordinary, routine, or broadly common aspects of existence from which the celebrated, dramatic, or rare have been excluded. The feature that defines the world of everyday life is not so much its familiarity, though it certainly is familiar, as it is the zone in which *my* life takes place, the zone in which *my* presence is actually located. Other realities (finite provinces of meaning) certainly exist as we all acknowledge, but this world of everyday life is my home. "It is impossible to overestimate the *centrality of the subject* for the phenomenal constitution of this world of everyday life" (Bittner 1973: 119–20).

Ethics has its fundamental reference to this historical and social world. This claim is a broadly Aristotelian view of ethics as a *practical* discipline that relies centrally on the exercise of moral judgment, rather than theoretical reasoning. Given the scope of the present study, however, I do not develop these important, but largely ancillary, philosophical concerns. The recent growth of applied ethics and bioethics attests to the growing philosophical recognition that ethics has an essential and not merely accidental connection with everyday life and its concrete problems. The analysis of ethical concepts or justification of ethical theory that had long been the main focus of philosophical ethics is now seen by various authors to have decisively turned to analysis of actual ethical dilemmas experienced in the everyday world (Jonsen and Toulmin 1988; Pincoffs 1986; Singer 1979; 1986; Williams 1985). Understanding the main lineaments and structural features of this world is, therefore, a prerequisite for dealing with the specialized ethical problems associated with long-term care.

The everyday commonsense world is the world of everyday life in which we carry out our day-to-day affairs. In this world we operate on the basis of typical or taken-for-granted ways of understanding and doing things. For example, in cooking a meal we engage in the doing itself. We are not usually reflectively concerned with where the food came from, how the electricity or gas used to cook the food was produced and delivered to us, or whether food producers and utilities producers are profiting. Instead, we are attentive to what immediately needs to be done: making sure the skillet is hot enough, finding the margarine, scrambling the egg, and so on. Even this brief description of a mundane event reveals how complex seemingly simple and routine activities are. Precisely because such activities are routinized, the world of everyday life conceals its internal complexity from us. We are engaged and live in this world and give our full attention to projects within it, but seldom do we withdraw to reflect on our activities and experiences. Instead, we are typically engaged in the world, simply busy with the many concerns and activities that make up our lives.

To speak of these activities as "routine" signifies that they are not only commonplace but also automatic or habitual, yet even this language—in part because of the prominence of the language of autonomy in our culture—is likely to be regarded as signifying something deficient and unfree. It should be easy to see that this bias is unfounded once we recall the discussion of human development in Chapter 4. The most routine and regular of our activities (indeed, activities that are not so much "active" but "automatic") are themselves the result of developmental achievement and effort that result from the reflexive interaction of the person as agent with the world. Importantly, a fully developed mature person, who is the ideal of liberal thought, is capable of rational decisionmaking precisely because, as an embodied self, one is able to rely unthinkingly on acquired habits and skills.

Consider, for example, the effort necessary for an adult to regain the ability to walk after an incapacitating injury. What is so easy, so mundane becomes for the individual in rehabilitation a matter of effort and striving. Each step involves a conscious exercise of the will to walk that confronts and must in some sense overcome a recalcitrant and resistant body. The need for effort and striving, basic elements of what autonomy developmentally involves, is everywhere in long-term care as elders are forced by their frailties and cognitive and physical incapacities to adapt and adjust themselves to the world.

As agents we function precisely on the basis of habits acquired historically. As the result of our development, we have at our disposal abilities that are layered one upon the other which we use without a bit of thought or consideration. This picture of the mature human person portrays developmental history as ever-present, automatically at one's disposal in the present. The underlying view of the person as agent in the world involves the recognition that human experience, despite the modern tendency to separate body and mind, is essentially embodied (Johnson 1987; Merleau-Ponty 1962; 1967). Actual autonomy involves considering not simply the mental processes of deliberation and choice in bodily action, but the function of the body in the mental processes themselves. To speak of autonomy in long-term care without attending to the bodily and experiential basis of meaning would make sense only on the basis of an abstract account that attended solely to idealized choice. Given the focus on actual autonomy in this work, such a gambit obviously is out of the question. Hence, consideration of some of the necessary conditions for concrete existence in the world is unavoidable.

Since development is never really completely past, it remains an essential possibility for even fully mature persons in the present. To be human is simply to have a future that is in a basic sense open, but always limited by the inevitability of death. When things fail to function, when things do not go right in the ordinary course of everyday experience, then we become aware, though sometimes only inchoately, of our nature as finite embodied persons. Encountering limitations, such as those imposed by illness, constitutes an important aspect of what Alfred Schutz termed "the fundamental anxiety" (1971a: 226–29). The experience of illness is the paradigm experience of the possibility of a fundamental disruption between the self and its being or existence in the world. We live in the world but we live, act, and experience the world as embodied creatures.

To be a person alive in the world thus necessarily entails an essential and ineliminable adhesion to the world. Hence to be free cannot, except on the basis of a convenient abstraction, mean that one is isolated and independently able to exercise a decision theoretic model of choice. Rather, to be concretely autonomous means that one has at one's disposal elements or features of one's own self that are presently not completely "free" precisely because they are not and cannot be contained within the scope of the rational choice or will. These aspects of the self are available *automatically* as acquired habit or skill. The practical problem of free choice is really a problem that must be set within the context of the world of everyday life. In this world, persons are free to act and choose as the liberal model would have it just because freedom is set within a context of acquired habits and formed identifications.

In the social world, experience can be described in terms of typifications, that is, the world is experienced not as a tissue of discrete impressions, but immediately as differentiated into "chairs," "animals," and "people" or, to be more precise, as "chairs which must be sold," "a room that appears strange and forbidding," and "friends who I will no longer see," or "strangers who come to care for me." In other words, things are experienced as typified within a broad context of actions, desires, and motives. This scheme of typifications, which sociologists speak of as constituting a "definition of reality," has important implications for the ethics of long-term care.

General Features of the Social Nature of Persons

To function as an agent in the social world requires that individuals have a broad set of abilities or skills, what has been termed a *stock of knowledge at hand*, that is acquired through habituation (Schutz 1970: 75–102, 133–62). The process whereby acquisition of basic skills necessary for agency occurs provides the empirical basis for the view of parentalism discussed in Chapter 2. This stock of knowledge at hand provides the foundation of our ability to act in the world. This general ability is made up of a variety of abilities that are developed over time and are layered or "sedimented" often in a complexly interdependent or hierarchical fashion. These abilities are not instinctual, but develop as individuals strive effortfully by acting in the world and through interaction with parents, peers, teachers, and others. To be an individual agent capable of independent action in the social world essentially requires relationships with others—others who necessarily figure in the development and sustenance of the abilities that allow an individual to be free. This point can hardly be overstressed.

The fundamental meaning of the autonomy of a person is thus bound up with that person's relationships with others: relationships with those who provided the nurturance that fostered the acquisition of basic motor and communication skills as well as those individuals who provide reinforcement and further development of skills throughout life. Acquiring skills and abilities to negotiate the social world is an essential ingredient in the development of a sense of self and mature personhood. In other words, to be a person, an autonomous moral agent, requires a prior relationship in which the fundamental processes of human growth and development can occur (Bowlby 1969; 1973; 1980; Spitz 1965). Far from being an isolated center of independent decisionmaking or action, human persons are agents in the everyday world precisely insofar as they are sustained by a complex web of interconnections and relationships with both past and present others. The concrete reality of human autonomy, therefore, bears little or no resemblance to the abstract picture provided by the liberal theory.

In order to function at all as agents in the world of everyday life, we regularly take a number of things for granted. We engage in actions and experience the world on the basis of *typifications*, that is, we simply assume that certain events or things are as they appear on the basis of past experience casting them as elements in one or another "ideal" category (type) that is part of our stock of knowledge at hand. Typifications serve their users by providing frames through which events are experienced and made meaningful. They do so by organizing expectations in a way that introduces a flexible ordering of the experiences of the world and its objects. As a corollary, typifications elaborate an understanding that allows us meaningfully to relate otherwise unconnected experiences or events. For example, the institutionalized elder experiences any caregiver as "nurse," a concept that indicates a generalized set of expectations regarding competence, knowledge, and function as well as expectations based on past experiences. Caregiving staff similarly typify elders in terms of disease categories or as "feeders," namely, those who need help eating. These terms denote rather heterogeneous classes that are nonetheless meaningfully associated in everyday experience. Such associations serve as practical guides to action by suggesting responses and expectations. Besides guiding action and organizing experience, typifications also have a profound rhetorical function, that is, to persuade and convince others about the proper interpretation of one's own and others' acts (Gubrium and Buckholdt 1977: 58–62). Typifications can thus either occlude intimacy or foster openness and trust in the other.

These functions of typifications collectively provide the means by which the everyday world is negotiated. *Negotiation* means to accomplish or cope with something, as in negotiating a sharp curve, and to arrange or settle by conferring or discussing with others, as when one negotiates a contract. Both aspects of the term are at work in the world of everyday experience as individuals interact both with the world and each other. We normally suspend doubt in the possibility that things might be otherwise than they appear. Doubt and disbelief, however, are intrinsic to human freedom, yet the everyday attitude suspends doubt and takes for granted that things are functioning as they are supposed to. As a result, we engage in activities in the everyday world until the taken-for-granted ways of doing things fail. These failures, problems, difficulties, and obstacles give pause to our engaged activity and occasion reflection. They force us to evaluate our situation which involves stepping back or disengaging from the world. Such disengagement is a prerequisite for reevaluation and choice and is a basic feature of the freedom of individuals that philosophers usually treat as if it were necessarily a high-order cognitive function. *Reflexion* rather than reflection seems to be what is required and occurs without the precision and clarity of the decision theoretic model of calculative choice.

To be an autonomous agent does not mean that, at bottom, one is independently self-sustaining and capable of critical reflective reasoning, but rather that the world as an object of experience is held in dynamic relationship by the intentional nature of consciousness itself. It is this dynamic power that is at the basis of the spontaneity that essentially comprises autonomy in its most basic form. Such a power underlies the capability of trying to (creatively) alter that involvement, an ability that often appears to be called forth by circumstances themselves and not initiated without them. Ironically, one common assumption of the traditional liberal view of autonomy is that it consists in the absence of obstacles when actual autonomy comes to the fore precisely when occlusions are encountered in daily living.

Frithjof Bergmann argued that the traditional concept of autonomy wrongly assumes both an absence of relationship and an absence of obstacles to choice or desire (1977: 41–53). The liberal view simply assumes that desire should hold sway no matter what. Everything, including social or ethical norms, historical and cultural circumstances, interpersonal relationships, or a myriad of other contingencies, must be swept aside on this view as autonomy expresses itself in the world. This view, however, is fundamentally mistaken. It is equally wrong to take the opposite view and argue that one is free not when there are no obstacles, because when there are no obstacles, failures, problems, or difficulties, one is simply busy, and so unreflectively bonded in habituated ways of involvement with the world and things. To be sure, only when routines break down, when normal expectations are frustrated, and when relationships come undone does reflection and conscious exercise of choice really enter, but these considerations are crucial only for autonomy regarded abstractly. Only an abstract account would regard the fecund experiences between the nodes of conflict or choice as nonfreedom. Of course, if one's model assumes that the person is primarily a rational decision maker and rationality is understood in intellectual terms, then the picture of someone fully engaged in action in the world unreflectively would surely seem strange. Yet the *strangeness* of this picture simply reveals the understandable, though not for that reason defensible, prejudice of typical philosophical treatments.

Despite the many kinds of frustration in our everyday experience of the world, we are usually able to attend sufficiently to practicalities so that we manage. For example, illness involving pain, confusion, distraction, depression, forgetfulness, and myriad other symptomatic alterations in consciousness deflect and distort the attention our everyday engagement in the world seems to demand. Even normal routinized activities become burdensome and difficult when illness or disability strikes because our basic bodily standing, our upright orientation in the world is affected (Straus 1963: 137–65). So-called coping strategies in effect usually involve utilizing or developing techniques to ameliorate the disengagement from the everyday world that illness or other experiences associated with daily living foist on us. Many of these dislocations are themselves fairly routine and expected; not surprising, we each possess various sets of techniques for adapting or coping.

The need to cope points out how central the social world of everyday life is to our very existence as human persons. We cope and adapt because we must get on with things, because we must engage in the world at hand. Reflection can be fruitfully regarded as the intellectual corollary of the wide range of adapting and coping behaviors that are routinely exhibited in daily life. It is the intellectual or cognitive expression of autonomy that presupposes the ability to disengage from involvement with, indeed, bondage to things in the everyday world. Reflection, however, occurs in the everyday world precisely when one's usual habits of thought or patterns of behavior are disrupted by either external or internal factors. What philosophers call *reflection* is primarily a disengaged, intellectual activity, namely, the critical or intellectual analysis and examination of ideas; this critical, intellectual activity is really a type of a much more common and variegated psychological process that is an essential feature of all human life. It is manifested in the everyday world in problem-solving and mundane, taken-for-granted decisionmaking about rather ordinary and unremarkable matters. To be autonomous, then, does not mean that one is simply free to choose in a vacuum, as it were, but to choose and act *in the midst of things*.

Explicit and self-aware reflection (as well as conscious or explicit choice) emerge from our daily interaction with the world and others. Infants are not born autonomous, but acquire freedom in the world as they develop skills and abilities that allow them to competently deal with the world (Haworth 1986). Hence, the phenomenological reality of human autonomy consists in its adherence to the world. Adherence is an important concept. By *adherence* I mean to suggest a relationship much like that of a plant enrooted in the earth. The earth does not hold it fast, but rather the plant through its root structure holds *itself* fast to the earth and draws nutrients therefrom. Similarly, the human person is bound to the world by the very nature of human existence and so the connection with the world is not one of bondage or enslavement, but of attachment. As the liberal theory would have it, autonomous relations of human persons with the world and with one another are misconstrued in a model that focuses on independence or negative freedom. To properly understand the nature of autonomy, then, it is necessary to take seriously the nature of human persons in their concrete involvement in the social world.

A significant feature of the social world of everyday life is that it assumes a common or shared culture (Garfinkel 1962). This common culture provides the taken-for-granted grounds for understanding and acting that make the everyday world a common or shared public world. This world is public in the sense that it is defined in terms of objective or clock time that makes common schedules possible (Zerubavel 1981); objective extension or space provides a reference in terms of defining your "there" and my "here" and it provides an orderly set of expectations for the way things happen in the world sequentially, one after another, or in joint occurrence and interaction. Sociologists have pointed out that this commonality of the social world involves shared beliefs and values that in a general way contribute to a broad range of expectations being experienced as "normal" or "usual." Such *typifications* are themselves the result of processes by which meanings and experiences are socially sedimented and become part of the common stock of knowledge on which mature persons acting in the world rely.

This observation is relevant for ethics since all practical reasoning arises from asking the question "What am I to do?" Asking that question, of course, has a point only when some reason has presented itself or been presented to the agent for doing something other than what is normal or typical. Good reasons for action, when they are effective in guiding action, are causes, and a cause is always something that makes a difference to an outcome. In human action the processes and procedures for which reasons for action make a causal difference are primarily those involving the everyday world with its schedule of routine activities. This concept of the normal day, month, year, and so on is of the first importance to understanding human action and reasoning about action in any culture. It is something in which philosophers have unfortunately shown remarkably little interest even though the structure of everyday normality provides the most basic framework for understanding human action.

Acting in accordance with the structures of the everyday world does not require that the agent be able to articulate reasons for acting, except in certain specific types of circumstance in which those structures have been put in question. Mundane necessities, such as meals eaten at certain prescribed times, in certain prescribed company, occur without anyone having to give reasons for doing so. In a similar fashion, work related to specific social roles or status occurs during scheduled periods; rituals occupy parts of the routinized day and reinforce the habits of structured activity. Both serious play and casual pursuits have their own structure and their own place in the larger structures (MacIntyre 1988: 24–25; Zerubavel 1981).

Acting for certain specific reasons is usually the exception. In normal circumstances, such "rational" action is intelligible only in terms of and against the background structures of everyday social normality. Action that departs from the background social expectations and norms is what usually requires that one have and be able to give reasons, typically for exemption from the tacitly accepted standards. What counts as an adequate or good reason for action is therefore first and foremost a reason good enough for doing something other than that which normality prescribes. The test of a good reason is not intellectual or formal rationality, but pragmatic rationality, namely, what works or what is accepted. Alasdair MacIntyre pointed out

> when a reason is judged to outweigh the requirements of the customary structure, there is in the background the possibility of a not-yet formulated judgment of some kind as to how good the reasons are for doing what the customary structure prescribes. And so reasoning which justifies particular requirements of that structure may emerge from the reasoning which puts it in question. But only in this secondary way do agents find reasons for doing what is normally prescribed. (1988: 25)

In point of fact, the structures of everyday normality serve primarily to make it unnecessary for most people most of the time to provide justifications for what they are doing or are about to do. Because most of what we do conforms to these general norms of everyday life, we are relieved of what would otherwise be an intolerable burden. This, of course, does not mean that the structures of the everyday world are transparent to understanding, but that for the agents involved they are mostly like the atmosphere, something on which we depend for life itself, yet completely unremarkable.

The person as agent in the everyday world is thus an essentially dependent entity, dependent on a socially derived stock-of-knowledge at hand and a repertoire of abilities and skills that comprise the background against which individual difference is manifested. In many respects, the focus on autonomy in ethics is best interpreted as a recognition or, indeed, an *insistence* on the importance of a sense of self, of individuality as a core concept for ethics, rather than as a claim for complete independence. That explains, in part, why many find the concept of autonomy to be a touchstone in ethics and medical ethics. The crucial issue is whether autonomy is theoretically understood in a thick or thin fashion, that is, whether the concept as theoretically articulated is sufficiently rich to endow autonomy with the substance and breadth it requires if it is to play the central role assigned to it in ethics. My earlier discussion of the liberal theory of autonomy was motivated by the belief that the typical expressivist account provides an inadequate or thin view of personhood, a view that is too narrow to support and sustain significant inquiry into the ethics of long-term care. A theory of autonomy that provides a concrete view of persons must be one that is sensitive to the social nature of personhood and to the complex conditions that actually support the unique identity of elders.

Adaptation to the social dislocation and physical disability and discomfort that usually precipitates the need for long-term care occurs within the social world, in the course of the elder's engaging or being unable to engage in daily living. Layered over these activities are the more complicated sets of emotional bonds to family and friends and those individual relationships that either continue in a modified fashion or are abated; thus, the insertion or presence, albeit altered, of even the frail or severely disabled elder in the social world is thorough. It could not, after all, be otherwise, yet the obvious is all-too-frequently forgotten. It is a fundamental mistake to regard individuals, even severely confused, withdrawn, or psychotic individuals, as somehow completely apart from the social world. Their involvement may be pathological and their existence in the social world may be deviant, precarious, or marginal at best—as judged from our standpoint, to be sure—but insofar as such individuals can be regarded as human persons in any minimal sense, they can be seen as functioning in the social world of everyday life.

Perhaps the best example of this point is the phenomenon of autism. Gerhard Bosch notes that one of the most striking features of autistic life consists in "positive peculiarities," which clearly point out what it means to be autistic:

> Once one has trained oneself to see these "positive peculiarities" of autistic children, it will be clear that they are extraordinarily attached to certain family situations, to being looked after by a certain person, and to a rigidly followed daily routine within which tenderness, such as a going-to-bed ritual with a good-night kiss and certain morning greetings, all have their place. These children are thus not just dependent and incapable of looking after themselves, but their whole behavior shows that they rely on and are adjusted to being cared for, dressed, fed, and looked after. Their behaviour presupposes the continued presence of someone to look after them, just like the small baby calling hungrily and searching with his mouth for the mother's breast. (1970: 59)

Even autistic life involves, according to Bosch, a kind of "symbiosis," a bond from which the individual partners cannot freely disassociate themselves without at once renouncing some or all of their own freedom (1970: 60). Thus, even at this developmental extreme, there is a social interdependence that sadly involves a form of attachment that assures a mature self will not emerge. At the other end of human development, however, illness-induced frailty need not mean abject dependence and isolation. If the impaired elder, moreover, is to sustain an identified sense of self, it must be cultivated and nurtured in the conditions that are necessary to sustain it. The calamity constantly lurking in the shadows of long-term care is that the sense of self in which autonomy actually resides will be forsaken.

An important point to stress is that the elder should not be regarded as completely or fully formed just because one is old. Persons are not completely made once and for all, but continue to develop throughout life. To be a person means to exist in dynamic tension and interaction with the world and others. Hence, to be a person is to never be fully complete or finished. In that sense, it is a mistake to think that caring for elders can involve only saving or preserving some remnant or trace of a past self. My analysis of the primacy of identification over free choice should not be taken to mean that we simply have to take the elder as we find her; that in some picayune sense the elder is simply who she is and that's that. The mature self is then not a finished product, but a subject who actively experiences the world on the basis of formed identifications. It is not over for the old just because they are old and frail; it is only over when, in fact, it is over, when death occurs.

As I argued in Chapter 4, the primacy of formed identifications concerns the meaning of the concept of autonomy and what it means to respect autonomy in the context of or with regard to the issue of choice. Here I am expanding the concept of autonomy to include the social nature of personal existence in the world of everyday life. A model that focuses exclusively on choice is inadequate because it misunderstands the primacy of identification, whereas a model that focused on identification as an accomplished fact would miss the developmental and socially interdependent nature of personhood. Elders are persons who are still engaged in that dynamic process of change through interaction with the world and others. It may be different, perhaps fundamentally so, from the development that marks the rest of the life span, but it is development as dynamic adaptation. The task, therefore, is not simply to preserve past identifications or some ideal state of functioning, but to find a richer and ethically more adequate way to conceptualize the features of the social world of everyday life of dependent elders across the entire range of human encounters in long-term care. Of the many features that might be explored, I focus on four themes that seem to play important roles in defining the autonomy of elders in long-term care: space, time, communication, and affectivity. Each are essential features of the world-making activity that is a corollary of autonomous engagement in the world of everyday life. Each theme proposes that autonomy in long-term care is largely an unrelenting effort to adapt to one's world, to find meaning as the body and mind suffer the pains and burdens of diminished capacities and limitations on experience.

Space

Space is not simply a geometric or mathematical construct that is objectively out there in the world. Rather, space must be understood as an aspect of human existence. The spatiality of human existence points to the openness and the availability of the person to the world. As Merleau-Ponty showed, the meaning of space is given to a person through that person's body (1962: 98–147). As one engages in different activities, one gears into the world and space takes on different meanings. For example, if one is playing golf, one might experience the course as something to be conquered or to be mastered. One must work both with and against its obstacles and traps. The course is thus a horizon for and object of attention and concentration. At the same time, the same space can be perceived as comfortable, a relaxing environment away from the stresses of work and family.

Similarly, space configures possibilities for movement and action. If one is impaired and wheelchair bound, then access is limited to surfaces conducive to the mode of conveyance. Also, one's perspective changes. We stand to face one another, to look one another "in the eyes." Yet, for the person in a wheelchair, eye level is at waist high for everyone else. In simplest terms, the body stands in a complex dialogue with the world primarily through movement or activity. Since space is not "objectively out there," but is a feature of human existence itself, human activities do not simply take place *in* space the way in which furniture fills a room or objects take up space on a shelf. The way a human being is in a space such as a room is through active interaction with the room and its contents. One can be in a room in a variety of ways, such as comfortably sitting in a chair while reading, in which case one's truly experienced space may well be "far away" in a fictional or phantasy world; or, one might be in a room alone and experience the room's emptiness and the temporary or even permanent absence of others; or, one might orient oneself toward the room as a project to be accomplished (walls to be painted, furniture to be rearranged, cleaning to be done).

The important implication of these points is that individuals requiring long-term care actively experience the world, but inevitably experience a distortion in the normal spatial relations that define the social world. If one does not leave one's apartment because one is not able, there is a significant diminishment of one's world. To be sure, this diminishment may be compensated by the use of a telephone, visitors, or letter writing and one's daily experience may be augmented by reading, watching television, and listening to the radio, but not *being able* to go out is different from not going out. The range of activity normally or typically open to frail elders is restricted. This diminishment is sometimes seen as a diminishment in the range of choice for the impaired elder, but such an interpretation is misleading. More important, the diminishment is itself a particular form of existence of elders, one that requires a compassionate and empathic understanding by caregivers. It is not simply a difference of degree, but of kind. The ethical question involves not the loss of independence or choice as such, but the loss of or threat to the self that restrictions in mobility may bring and the meaning of the new perception of space. Restrictions in mobility invariably bring modifications in the experience of space, modifications that require the individual to adapt.

Observational research regularly points to the importance of time and space as components structuring nursing home existence (Savishinsky 1991: 188–90). The very architecture of nursing homes tends to reflect and serve the convenience of the staff and their work routines. Disease has already disabled the elder; now strange noises, rhythms, and procedures in the nursing home further enfeeble and baffle. The sick elder is removed from a familiar setting where they feel in charge into a setting in which strangers assume control. No wonder that elders balk, even more than others who are sick, at entering total institutions. The stakes are so much higher for them. Sick people normally go to the hospital because they have no alternative and they have reasonable hope to come out alive, but for a significant number of elders the move into institutional care is permanent. The institution swallows them up in its own rhythms and impersonal and unfamiliar space. Limited room prevents elders from bringing many of their valued possessions and other tokens of identity. The new location often removes them from their communities; in effect, they are condemned to a kind of premature burial.

> Successively and progressively, impairment, old age, immobility, and death restrict space. The world at large shrinks to a single room and ultimately to a casket. Ordinarily, people live in a number of different environments—home, workplace, streets, parks, gardens, and sidewalks. The bedroom is only part of a total world, often a sanctuary from it. But, for the immobile or the impaired, the world contracts to a single room. Designers of total institutions take on an awesome responsibility. They create for residents not just a fragment but the whole of their perceivable world. (May 1986: 46)

J. H. van den Berg described how confinement to a bed during illness establishes a new world for the patient (1966). After several days the bed begins to smell, the odors of cloth, bed sheets, covers, pillows, and pajamas become an intimate part of the limited world of the sick person. The existence of the individual becomes vapid and stale as the patient slips into passivity and dependence. Since things must be done by others, the individual loses physical contact not only with the surroundings, but also with one's own body. Daily hygiene and other activities of daily living are taken over by others; as a result, one's usual privacy is lost. Losing a sense of intimate or private space for these necessary functions brings forth an experience of shame that is not circumscribed by others, but spills over into oneself toward one's body. As a result, it seems that nothing is left to the person. It is as if one has "abdicated" whole portions of the self. The experience of shame and enforced inactivity manifests itself in a psychological distancing from the external world and one's own body.

> The sick estrange themselves, even from their own bodies. In this way the bed reinforces the dis-ease that has placed them there. In a literal sense sick persons can no longer be sure of themselves, can no longer recognize themselves through their usual posture, their customary and characteristic movements. They can no longer reconnoiter space; they can no longer make conquests something that would contribute to their sense of wholeness. Space becomes something alien, unconquerable, no longer to be used. (Bergsma and Thomasma 1982: 131)

As embodied, we define our relationship to the world actively through what Erwin Straus termed *the upright posture* (1966: 137–65). The upright posture is widely recognized as a significant evolutionary development for the human species. In philosophical terms the upright posture signifies the orientation of humans to the world, an orientation that defines a uniquely human existence. That existence is an existence in essential tension with the world. Spatially, humans exist in a vertical dimension that defies gravity and defines the world as a horizontal field for action. The idea of movement itself implies a functional relationship between human vital relations and values, between behavior and circumstances, between position and a sense of place, between action and things in the world. Hence, it is no wonder that for the sick or impaired elder, normal realities are to a great extent experienced as cramped and remote or as simply alien; the disabled elder, especially one without significant or meaningful social contacts and interactions, thus naturally focuses on her own bodily processes or on the bed—a very narrow and limited horizon indeed. The attention to "bed and body" work by caregivers instead of to the person receiving the care insinuates a sense of isolation reinforcing and confirming a sense of being lost or confused.

One kind of consequence of the changes in spatial perception and experience brought on by illness that engender long-term care is that personal and intimate matters become hardly experienced as such and, in an important sense, are abdicated by the sick person. Rather than *being* a body, the sick elder finds that he or she simply *has* a body (Marcel 1965). Others care for the body as they will, not as the elder wills. Bergsma and Thomasma similarly described the distancing that occurs between the body and the self as the prone body is constrained in an unnatural horizontal position (1982: 130–34). Whether constrained horizontally or in a gerichair or wheelchair, the impaired elder exists in a severely limited environment. The environment is limited not just de facto, because in a sense anyone can at any point in time just happen to be in a relatively confined space, but as an essential condition; for the elder requiring long-term care, confinement is an essential feature of existence.

The normal or typical proportions of reality are altered both through the illnesses and disabilities that elders in long-term care suffer and by the social and physical structure of long-term care itself. It is not simply that the environment or setting changes as an elder moves from an upstairs bedroom to a first-floor living room, from an apartment into a child's home or an institutional long-term care setting, or from custodial to skilled care within a nursing home, but the significance and meaning of those changes of scene are just as pregnant with possibilities and fraught with peril as scene changes in a murder mystery. These changes are significant because the person's fundamental experience of space is altered and, in some instances, curtailed. Perceptual distortions occur as the result of illness. As time goes on, the body itself becomes a part of the truncated environment. It becomes an object from which the self is dispossessed. Even in home care, the home becomes less "homey" and more foreign or strange as it mutates from the place where one lived actively into the place where one receives care. Obviously, the kinds of care received and the perceptual meaning of the home space for the elder before and during home care are unique to the particular individual and circumstance.

While space is an essential feature of human experience in the everyday world, it is not an abstract or generic element. Space, along with other dimensions of autonomy in the everyday world, has particular and specific meanings. These dimensions are features of the ambient environment that sustain the life of individual persons. It would be as absurd to speak of the spatial needs of an elder in long-term care abstractly as it would be to speak of the needs of a particular species of fish, but fail to consider that the "space" of the fish is a watery world. In nursing homes, however, such mistakes are frequently made. When an elder leaves a nursing home for a brief hospitalization, it is not uncommon to find that their old room was reassigned during their absence and that they were temporarily or permanently moved to another area of the home. Apparently, nursing homes observe their contractual responsibilities by providing an abstract "space" rather than a particular room or bed, forgetting that not all rooms and beds are meaningfully the same to the elder. This insensitivity strikes one as analogous to the failure to remember the need for water (of a certain temperature, pH, or clarity) for a particular species of fish.

Implications for Long-Term Care

The ethical implications of this analysis involve questioning how practices associated with long-term care (1) identify these features and (2) deal with their impact on the elder's sense of autonomy and self-worth. Does long-term care actually impose unreasonable and unwarranted limitations on what is already a truncated existence or is it designed to compensate for or to accommodate altered experience and need? In a sense, it almost seems perverse to worry about independence and choice in a circumstance in which there seems to be very little actual independence or prospect thereof and very little about which to exercise effective or meaningful choice. If I am not free because I am not able even to move about, if barriers exist at every turn, or if I am unable even to turn myself in bed, then it seems that my very being as a human person is fundamentally altered insofar as the basic spatial dimension of existence is radically restricted. The restriction at issue here is neither simply imposed by others nor simply a limitation imposed on one's physical life space, but rather those changes in the basic *experience* of space (cf. Bachelard 1969) and the possibility of meaningful action for the elder.

The difficulty is related to our traditional failure to grasp the essential connections between motility, sentience, and emotion. As Hans Jonas expressed it:

> Locomotion is toward or away from an object, i.e., pursuit or flight. A protracted pursuit . . . bespeaks not only developed motor and sensor faculties but also distinct powers of emotion. It is safe to assume that the number of intermediate steps over which the purpose can extend itself is a measure of the stage of emotional development. . . . It is motility which makes the difference [between sheer maintaining of metabolism and genuine appetition] visible: it consists in the interposition of *distance* between urge and attainment, i.e., in the possibility of a distant goal. Its apprehension requires distant perception: thus development of sentience is involved. Its attainment requires controlled locomotion: thus development of motility is involved. But to experience the distantly perceived *as* a goal and to keep its goal quality alive, so as to carry the motion over the necessary span of effort and time, desire is required. Fulfillment not yet at hand is the essential condition of desire, and deferred fulfillment is what desire in turn makes possible. Thus desire represents the time-aspect of the same situation of which perception represents the space-aspect. (1966: 101)

Failure to inform the analysis of long-term care with these points is a natural corollary of an abstract approach to autonomy. The advantage afforded by these points is readily apparent. For example, the elder with impaired motor and sensory faculties thus naturally experiences a diminution in her world. Spatially, the world is not only objectively smaller but subjectively contracted; it is experienced more as a closed space than as an open space that invites activity. It seems hardly surprising that, given the problems that bring patients into institutionalized care, wandering or confusion is such a prominent behavior. Such individuals are simply lost— lost in a strange world and lost to themselves. This behavior is not to suggest, much less argue, that wandering or confusion cannot have physiological causes, but rather that in human terms the loss of a world that is open for meaningful action constitutes a fundamental assault on the very nature of being a human person. As a result of this assault, individuals feel lost; they do not know their way about. Since these individuals are still mobile, they naturally move about, yet their movement is apparently meaningless, without direction or explicit purpose. Physiological causation aside, the significance of these changes as fundamental distortions in the very quality of space itself is experienced by elders as they interact with the world. Wandering and confusion, then, would best be regarded as phenomena that solicit the concerned involvement of caregivers rather than as phenomena that call for "management" and "control," because these phenomena can possibly be related to fundamental distortions in the elders' experienced sense of space brought about by elders' (possibly ineffectual) effort to deal with the motor and sensory impairments that cause them to need long-term care in the first place (Demitrack and Tourigny 1988).

Although the idea of a personal space has been a contentious subject in psychological research (Hayduk 1983; Mishra 1983), it is clear that space has psychological significance for persons. The significance requires exploration in particular cases, but the absence of sensitivity to this area of concern is evident in practices such as allocating rooms and roommates in nursing homes (Miles and Sachs: 1990). One's sense of self, of personal integrity, involves a certain sense of privacy and personal space. We *are* in a significant and irreducible sense both our body and the space we inhabit. The identification at stake here is perhaps the most fundamental, yet remarkably inchoate. Nursing home existence unfortunately appears to intensify, rather than ameliorate, the violation of personal privacy and space that elders experience as the consequence of their physical impairments. Each resident has a "chart" with a "history" that is available to all staff, but largely a mystery to the elder herself. Facts about the patient that may not be exhibited at present, but are known to the staff, become factors in decisions, for example, to restrict an elder's movements as a way to protect the elder (Priester 1990; also, see illustrative cases in Kane and Caplan 1990).

The importance of space in social life generally and nursing home experience is the subject of a growing literature (Altman 1975; Brent 1984; Koncelik 1976; Lawton 1981; Lawton, Liebowitz, and Charon 1970; Moos and Igra 1980; Moos and Lemke 1979; 1980; Ohta and Ohta 1988; Sommer 1969). Uriel Cohen and Gerald D. Weisman (1990) argued that interest in the therapeutic potential of the physical environment starting with Kleemeier (1959) has grown during the last two decades to the point where it is now possible to place the concept of autonomy in its proper environmental context. They identify three environmental aspects of autonomy: mobility and independence, control and freedom of choice, identity and continuity that support a set of two dozen principles for the design of environments for people with dementia (Cohen and Weisman 1991).

One practical implication of these reflections on the positive aspects of space in the experience of the confused or cognitively impaired elder is on the widespread problem of wandering. The use of physical restraint is a common practice in the institutional care of elders who wander, appear abusive, or are so frail that they are considered likely to fall (Evans and Strumpf 1989). Apparently, many institutions believe that the use of physical restraints is the most effective way to protect elders, even though restraining comprises an egregious restriction on autonomy as negative freedom. Response to wandering behavior is sometimes achieved through high tech devices like electronic alarms or, in the extreme, "harness systems" that tether residents to lines suspended from overhead trolleys (Colvin 1989). Employment of these devices is justified by appeal to the need to protect the safety of wandering and confused elders. The conflict between autonomy as independence and free movement on the one hand and protection of the physical well-being of the elder on the other is starkly evident.

Frequently, institutions report that they are motivated to restrain patients by fear of lawsuit. However, as of 1989, no lawsuit has yet been successful against a facility solely for failure to restrain a resident (Blakeslee, Goldman, and Papougenis 1990: 80). The risk of liability for false imprisonment, assault, or injury or death from restraint is much greater with misuse of physical restraints (Blakeslee, Goldman, and Papougenis 1990: 80). Indeed, studies of two communities that do not use restraints indicate that they have no more injuries from falls than do facilities that employ such devices (Blakeslee, Goldman and Papougenis 1990: 80). To replace physical restraints, however, requires adopting individualized, humane approaches to care. Experience shows that use of restraints actually requires more staff than less because immobilization causes chronic constipation, pressure sores, loss of bone mass, muscle atrophy, decreased ability to ambulate, and eventual invalidism (Miller 1975; Warshaw, Moore, Friedman, *et al.* 1982). The use of alarms on the doors to elders' rooms and on exit doors, placement of yellow barrier strips fastened by Velcro, or use of a mat at the threshold of a doorway help deter some confused patients from entering or leaving areas. They do so by providing perceptual cues that afford elders choices to proceed or alter their movement. More staff are not necessarily required to permit elders this kind of freedom of movement; only a commitment that staff from every department are responsible for wandering elders and that caregivers share one-on-one supervision during times when an elder is particularly anxious. The goal is to make the environment as safe as possible by being sensitive to the *purposeful* routine of wandering behavior, not by removing all risk.

Key to a restraint-free approach in the care of the wandering and confused elder seems to involve a conceptual change on the part of caregivers. Staff are required to depart from normal "bed and body" work and engage in examining problem situations and actively work toward resolving the particular problem by attempting to understand the meaning latent in the seemingly purposeless movement of the cognitively impaired elder. Clearly, a significant conceptual change is required before this kind of approach can be adopted, though its rationale and justification are squarely located in the positive view of autonomy as identification. Maintaining mobility and independence involves more than simply assuring safety and security, but consists as well in eliminating environmental barriers that provide opportunities for meaningful wandering. If wandering is not viewed as a problem to be controlled, but is an opportunity to engage individuals in actions that occur along well-defined, secure, and engaging paths, then the wandering behavior of the cognitively impaired elder can permit mobility and independence to occur (Cohen and Weisman 1990: 76).

The spatial environment plays an important role in controlling elders or enhancing their choice and range of experience. Electing protection without considering the costs to the quality of experience of the cognitively impaired elder is to thwart rather than respect the elder's autonomy. Coons (1987) suggested that rigid schedules and hospital-like design elements are not suitable for long-term care, particularly for residents who are cognitively impaired. The desideratum is an environment that affords opportunities to choose from among a variety of spaces, from private to public. Such choice facilitates elders' control of both their sensory and social stimulation and may reduce the perceived intrusion into or threat to their own individual space. Finally, the importance of identification, as discussed earlier, provides a positive and practical ground for enhancing a range of meaningful choices for the confused and cognitively impaired elder. As Cohen and Weisman put it:

> To the extent that individuals have the opportunity to make meaningful decisions about their environments, they can maintain ties to their past lives. . . . For people with dementia, familiar artifacts, activities, and spaces can provide valuable personal associations and can stimulate opportunities for social interaction and meaningful activity. Rather than being limited to a single "rummage box," the total environment may be utilized to trigger reminiscence. (1990: 76)

Time

The second element comprising the world of everyday life that is important for autonomy and long-term care is the temporal aspect of existence. As with space, time is not simply an objective dimension in which human beings hapto exist and find themselves. Rather, temporality is an essential feature of being human (Minkowski 1970); it is also an important concern of gerontologists (Hendricks and Hendricks 1976; Kastenbaum 1963; 1969a; 1975; 1977; Moody 1984a; 1984b).

Humans are essentially temporal; they come into being and develop as persons in time and constitute their identities historically. As pointed out earlier, humans develop as persons only through their participation in a social world. Thus, relationships with others are necessary both for a sense of self and a sense of world. To properly interpret autonomy, then, we must consider the temporal aspect of human existence not simply as a frame for choice or decisionmaking, but as an existential and social matrix against which the very concept of something as a project is possible (Schutz 1970: 67–96).

The notion that there is an objective time "out there" is itself a feature of the everyday world. We act *as if* time existed objectively. One way that we orient ourselves in the social world, the world of action and work, is through timepieces. Reckoning time is one way to establish a sense of reality even in strange or unfamiliar surroundings because it reestablishes oneself in that one dimension that assures social continuity, the shared dimension of time. Gubrium, too, reported that elders at Murray Manor often commented on or asked each other and staff what day it was; careful tracking of time, however, occurred mostly when the elder had a scheduled appointment outside the nursing home, though some kept track of clock time in order to watch favorite television programs (1975: 169). Shared time helps define not only the social world of action and work, but a fundamental orientation as well. In the social world, individuals go about the myriad activities that comprise their day-to-day existence. Whatever modifies that existence (e.g., illness or a special event such as a marriage, holiday, or death of a friend or loved one) has an effect on the experience of time, namely, the typical ebb and flow of events is temporally deformed and shaped by the significance of the events. Nursing home life, judging from the ethnographic literature, seems to have no fundamentally shared sense of time, except for the depersonalized institutional regimen. As a result, elders seem adrift; no wonder that confusion is such a commonly reported finding, since the basic temporal structure of reality orientation in the everyday world is itself experientially distorted.

People active in their day-to-day lives often do not have enough time. They are busy with many things, and many interests compete for their attention. Alterations in their schedule either slow down or speed up the sense of passing time and give time a heavy or a light feeling. When I say I don't have time for something, I deny, in a sense, that thing its importance or value. When I make time for something, I focus my attention on it, and so include that thing within my existence in anticipation and projectively. A child or spouse who complains that the father working constantly does not have time for her is complaining about the way that she feels devalued by the father's inattention or preoccupation with other things, even while the father might actually spend time in her presence. The child or spouse may complain: the father is not really *here* in the very time purportedly spent together! Time spent with the preoccupied father goes too quickly or does not afford the sense of openness because it seems that preoccupation with work intrudes not only on the details of the relationship, but its temporal quality as well.

Similarly, an institutionalized elder might employ various techniques to solicit attention designed to bring staff members or others into her temporal world so as to force them to make time for herself, not simply as a patient needing professional or technical care but as a person needing the attention of other humans (Gubrium 1975: 158–96). It is important to distinguish the tasks performed or services rendered from care that is manifested with concern. One can adequately provide a service without due regard for the person receiving it, without affective or emotional engagement, but care necessarily requires engagement and engagement involves people tuning into one another's temporal stream "making music together" (Schutz 1971b: 159–78).

Patients commonly complain about caregivers or praise them on the basis of their refusal or willingness to spend time with them. Indeed, one wonders why time spent together is so important to elders, especially in nursing homes. Given that one's feelings or sense of reality is always confirmed or disconfirmed by others, especially authority figures, in the social world, when elders experience staff members as not having time for them, as failing to acknowledge or affirm that their needs and suffering are real, it is not surprising that the elders would feel devalued and depersonalized, even though the services rendered are objectively good. Too often, it seems, staff members are unwilling or unable to acknowledge the suffering and isolation of patients because they feel incapable of doing anything effective to correct or ameliorate it, yet patients sometimes want only the social affirmation that their suffering and loneliness are precisely theirs. For their suffering to be truly their own, it must be shared with others. Hence, patients seek or demand attention from staff members or others less out of an idiosyncratic need than as an essential human requirement. Being a witness to such experience or, more actively said, *giving* witness, seems to be quite foreign to health care professionals, who go about their daily business officiously performing caregiving tasks.

The dimension of time in the nursing home as a workplace for staff and as an everyday life context for patients can be radically different, though the importance of temporal features of social institutional life is a relatively new research theme (Zerubavel 1979; 1981).

As Alfred Schutz suggestively observed:

> It appears that all possible communication presupposes a mutual tuning-in relationship between the communicator and the addressee of the communication. This relationship is established by the reciprocal sharing of the Other's flux of experiences in inner time, by living through a vivid present together, by experiencing this togetherness as a "We." Only within this experience does the Other's conduct become meaningful to the partner tuned in on him—that is, the Other's body and its movements can be and are interpreted as a field of expression of events within his inner life. . . . Communicating with one another presupposes, therefore, the simultaneous partaking of the partners in various dimensions of outer and inner time—in short in growing older together. This seems to be valid for all kinds of communication. (1971b: 177–78)

If this observation is correct, then the importance of time in establishing a common and shared world and in making possible genuine communication becomes apparent. The failure of caregivers to "tune-in" to elders deprives elders of participation in the process of "growing older together," a failure due, perhaps, to health professionals own psychological defenses against death and dying. The net effect, however, is that elders, by being excluded, are treated as if they existed outside shared human time—as if they were dead already. Thus, for the elder to truly belong to a world, the elder must be allowed to share time with significant others. Allowing this to occur, then, would seem to be a significant way to respect the frail elder as a person.

A component of time that has important implications for autonomy is the meaning of scheduled time for the elder. The more important or central a block of time or the activity ongoing during that time is to an individual, the more important it is whether the time is self-scheduled and controlled or other-scheduled and controlled (Gubrium 1975: 158–96; Zerubavel 1981). Our basic orientation to the world of everyday life is in terms of normal activities and rituals such as basic tasks of daily living that inevitably have a particular rhythm and schedule. Modifications in such schedules or rhythms, either drastic as in the regimented total environment of a nursing home or changes due to the availability of a home care provider, pose conflicts and problems for elders. Since one basic mark of status and power is the ability to control or adapt one's own schedule of activities, modifications owing to caregiver needs represent more than marginal impacts on elder autonomy.

One of the most important and perhaps the deepest philosophical problem associated with autonomy in long-term care is the effacement of a social and personal sense of self through psychological and physical disability brought on by diseases associated with aging and the inevitability of death. Rational choice is future oriented. It chooses between alternatives available in the present in order to achieve outcomes in the future. The temporality of human existence makes this circumstance a necessity. Of course, one can also choose a past. It may seem surprising but people work at reconstituting who they are or have been in the past. The past is not somehow preserved "in reality" or objectively; the past is, like the future, indeterminate for humans.

Consider history. Does historical research uncover past "facts" that are there objectively to be discovered or is history a complex process of human interpretation, involving the reconstitution and reconstruction of a sense of the past? To be sure, empirical evidence plays an important role, but so do present historically and socially conditioned attitudes and beliefs that influence the selection and interpretation of the "relevant" facts. This means that "the" past is an idealization, which is constantly in change as we reflect historically and as we move as historical creatures into our own future (Collingwood 1959).

What is true for the discipline of history is also true for individuals. One is always in dynamic interaction with one's past as well as with the present and future. The past needs work if it is to be preserved as one's past at least for the simple reason that without reflection and recollection the past ceases to be a distinctively human past. Events, persons, interactions, and other things of importance are forgotten, their significance altered unless actively maintained. In part, various social rites and rituals surrounding family gatherings, for example, both recollect and reconstitute the past for new sons-in-law and daughters-in-law, for new children and grandchildren in the family, as well as for each family member.

The family is an important provider of care for the frail or disabled elder in America (Uhlenberg 1987). This fact points to deep-seated bonds of affection and commitment that need explanation. Temporally, these bonds are constituted not in terms of some future benefit, some rational decision regarding what is appropriate or best given circumstances, but on the basis of what is "right," "proper," or "appropriate" based on who we are; who we are is based on whom we have become in the past. The past thus exerts an important but not a deterministic influence on all of us; it gives us a basis and a foundation for movement into the uncertainty of the future. The past provides the basis for our present and future responsibilities. On its basis, we have a whole set of skills, recipes for action or typifications that enable us to function in the social world. Included with these typifications are emotional bonds or beliefs that involve the trust (or mistrust) that individuals have in one another and in their own abilities. One problem with the traditional model of autonomy is that it assumes that individuals are isolated. They exist in an atemporal "eternal now" contemplating the implications and consequences of their actions in an indeterminate future in terms of costs and benefits. But for choices to appear *as choices*, that is, as choices not in some logical sense, but choices that are experienced as *real* choices or real options for an individual, they must cohere with patterns of expectation developed in the past.

The human mind cannot function if it is overwhelmed by options whose variety is either so great or whose novelty cannot be readily assimilated into the person's frame of reference. Instead, a choice is a choice because it *means* something to a chooser. It means something either in the sense of something desirable, undesirable, or at least something sensible as an alternative. Truly new alternatives are

often not experienced by individuals as real alternatives just because the very new-
ness of the choice at hand precludes it from being experienced as a meaningful
option. Hence, we choose and enact a future because we have a past that vitally
structures our experience of the world. Without a past, cut off from our own
resources, our own skills and habits of thought, we are bereft of the ability to function as an agent.

Losing agency is more fundamental than losing the opportunity to choose. To
lose agency does not mean that we cannot indicate a preference from among a
range of options, but rather that such indication will lack meaning for us. For
example, consider an everyday experience. A person is bored and lonely sitting in
front of a television with a remote control channel changer. It would be descriptively inaccurate to say that *she* flits from one channel to another; rather, it is the
television that presents one option after another in rapid succession. It is not true
that none of the programs available satisfies her entertainment desires, but that
none of this will do because something more—whatever that might be—is wanted.
Hence, even though the individual might settle on a particular channel and a particular program, it does not indicate that meaningful choice was exercised and that
the program chosen was significant for the individual. Quite the contrary, when
alternatives are not experienced as meaningful to individuals' core identifications,
boredom comes to the fore. Individuals defend their sense of self from meaningless choices by either complaining that no choice is available which is literally
true in the sense of no "real," "true," or "meaningful" choice or they passively
submit to whatever comes their way since none of it matters anyway.

This loss of meaning even in the face of objective evidence of "choice" is an
important phenomenon with which the traditional model of autonomy is ill-equipped
to deal. Why is this so? In part, because the traditional model of autonomy ignores
the historical and social nature of human existence. We have discussed this already
in some detail. In a sense, the model is primarily concerned that freedom of choice
or preference not be impaired or interfered with by others, but is not particularly
concerned that the choices available are meaningful. There is, however, another
implication, namely, that in ignoring the historical and temporal character of human
existence, the traditional model—and those reforms motivated by its rhetoric—
has no way of making sense of hope.

Individuals in long-term care, at least those who require intensive nursing care
but perhaps also those who require only custodial support, frequently have relatively little of importance to make choices about. Defenders of the traditional model
of autonomy often forget this compelling point. To underscore and stress choice
in a circumstance in which viable alternatives are personally meaningless or un-
important seems either absurd or cruel. Yet, the reality of long-term care for many
is precisely a situation in which there are no particularly meaningful choices. What
then is to be done? This question cannot be answered simply by thinking in a more
fine-grained approach about alternatives because the critical point is that the options, no matter how many more are made available can never be made meaningful by the same strategy that increases the range of choice. We simply have to
look in a different direction.

Implications for Long-Term Care

Since humans are temporal beings, they exist in time and must apportion their attention and, in so doing, themselves. One of the basic exercises of autonomy involves the bestowal of one's attention. Caregivers, either busy nursing assistants or reluctant family members, who do not have time for elders do have time for other things and those other things are shown to be more important than the elders. Requests by a dependent elder that go unanswered are valued differently from other activities, such as maintaining records or carrying on with other activities in the home. The irony here is that choices must be made. It is surprising that staff members often are quick to note and complain that old people live in the past, not the present or do not look forward to things—though it is hard to see what one has to look forward to in many long-term care settings—but they often forget that they too go about their daily activities of caregiving in such a routinized fashion that it permits them to dwell temporally elsewhere. For example, one can meet the bodily needs of patients, the "bed and body work" (Gubrium 1975: 123–57), with a degree of disengagement that permits the caregiver to save the real time for oneself. That is, insofar as activities are routinized or delivered without due interaction, they demand less of the self and allow the self to fantasize, to daydream, to sustain a psychic distance from those ostensible subjects of caregiving. Similarly, the distancing of elders from their surroundings and caregivers in nursing homes can partly be attributed to the imposition of institutional time regulation on their already truncated existence.

Erving Goffman's classic discussion of the total institution focuses on the regulation of normal activities (1960; 1961). One way in which these activities are regulated is through structuring time. Of course, time is structured everywhere in the social world, probably less so for individuals who are unemployed and engaged in housework activities than for people in the workplace, but since humans exist in the social world, they exist in a structured temporal order. That order makes sense because it makes possible certain typified kinds of activity. It regularizes the routines of the toilet, bathing, dressing, eating, and working. That order also regularizes our relationships with one another, even intimate relationships with our loved ones. These ordered structures are not fixed and rigid, but they define a pattern in terms of which individuals organize their lives and expectations in the social world. Notice, however, that when one's horizon of action diminishes, the given or usual ordered structure of time is correspondingly altered.

Consider a vacation. One can sleep in. One can lunch early or late. One can engage in leisure reading or sports in what would normally be the work day. One has time for significant others. Indeed, families who vacation together and limit sightseeing and organized activities can reestablish a sense of intimacy and belonging that often recedes in the workaday world. Holidays have a similar function. Time in institutional long-term care and even in home care settings is structured differently from that in most social settings, no doubt partly because elders are relatively disengaged from the more structured demands of the workaday world. Truly engaged caregiving is time intensive. Caregivers, particularly family caregivers, also require time away from the primary site to reestablish their own sense of meaningful identifications.

In the home setting, caregiving activities can occur spontaneously according to an individual and organically derived schedule, but often have to become routinized according to the schedule of the visiting home care provider or the family caregiver because of other commitments, not the elder. In an institutional setting, temporal organization becomes far more extensive and often more rigid. As an individual ages and withdraws from the work world and limits social activities, she gains a freedom from the burdens of socially determined schedules. In a sense, an elder gains time, even as one is losing time because of the approach of death. In institutional care, however, the bureaucratic structure imposes a different temporal structure on the basic rhythm of daily life, a structure that is geared toward the workaday world of the staff more than to the needs of patients. When patients are awakened, bathed, and dressed or put to bed is usually determined more by staffing requirements and the change of shifts than by sensitivity to the preferences or expectations of the elders themselves. I am not suggesting that the bureaucratic nature of most institutional care, especially the temporal organization of caregiving, is ethically problematic in itself, but that the temporal organization and structure of an institution should not simply be accepted without question, but should itself be subject to scrutiny regarding its effect on promoting and respecting the autonomy of elders.

If time defines the nature of social reality, then the temporal dimension of existence must be seriously considered. If I cannot sleep and have nothing else to do, I am left with ennui. Ennui may itself be a significant source of patient fatigue; boredom simply means that one is experiencing an emptiness between structured events in time, events in time structured by others and out of one's control (Bergsma and Thomasma 1982: 138–40). Elements that are typically structured in our society include going to work, eating meals, and making arrangements that often accompany meal preparation and meal time. In addition, persons structure their lives around special social events, such as weddings, as well as the more usual, but nonetheless personally meaningful activities, such as the chance to finish reading a good book, to clean the garage, or to shop without the children. For bedfast, institutionalized elders or elders with restricted mobility, few of these personally structured events are actually available, especially since these elders frequently suffer from cognitive disorders or confusion. Instead, the institutional schedule and structure takes over and the patient is oriented instead toward waking up, washing, meals, and lights out. Hence, it is no wonder that patients attach unusual significance to these institutional routines. Ask a patient to describe the day, and the description will usually focus on when he awoke, when he bathed, when he ate, and whether he slept well or not (Bergsma and Thomasma 1982: 138–39).

Since there is nothing else to occupy the patients' time, since they have usually nothing to "do," time hangs over them like a burden. Pacing back and forth, waiting for coffee, and eating are activities that significantly occupy patients, yet these activities cannot really be regarded as intentional, since they are not actually structured and productive in the normal sense. As a result, patients may complain about fatigue; such fatigue might result from the unintentional nature of much of what they do each day. When one is really engaged in work, one seldom feels tired or at least does not significantly experience fatigue during the activity. That comes later.

Complaints about fatigue are often an escape. Bergsma and Thomasma suggested that fatigue is relatively similar to regression in the sense that both can be seen as attempts to escape, not from the situation as such but from the feeling of being conquered by it (1982: 139). This sense of being conquered and out of control indicates how elders in long-term care are blocked from the paramount reality of the social world and isolated from their own sense of agency and self-worth. Since they have nothing to do or since they are not able or not permitted to do what they themselves see as important, they engage in apparently meaningless motions that can hardly be called activities in the sense of being the intentional production of an agent. Behind the observational facade of purposelessness, there is a good deal of effort and work by elders to cope with the time that is left in their hands.

Observational studies of institutional elders, for example, report that even seriously compromised and cognitively impaired elders actively work, indeed, struggle to fill up their time (Diamond 1986; Gubrium 1975). Elders engage in various activities that seem designed to pass time or to fill up time with some meaningful activity or experience. This is not a continuous activity, but is divided up, like the institutional day, into three parts by meals (Gubrium 1975: 161–68). The institutionally imposed structure of time is, of course, designed around the needs of the staff, not the needs or interests of elders, many of whom complain about scheduled meal, sleep, or wake-up times. As Eviatar Zerubavel (1979) has pointed out, there are strikingly stable and elaborate temporal patterns and structures in the everyday work world of the hospital; it is not surprising that these patterns and structures are evident in long-term care as well.

These observations, however, do not imply that agency is simply absent; autonomy is present but its modality is radically altered. Time is crucial both for deciding and choosing courses of action as well as executing those choices. There are important linkages between the temporal dimension of everyday life and phenomena such as reminiscence and reconstructing biography observed in elders (Johnson 1976; Merriam 1980). Reminiscence and telling stories about one's life is not dwelling in the past, a refusal to live in the present and a withdrawal, but involves psychological processes related to adapting oneself to new circumstances. Reconstructing biography and telling stories of one's life are integrative efforts leading to an overall intelligibility. Identifying who one is, not conceptually or analytically by declaring one's values and beliefs, but narratively through stories about oneself is a common way of establishing orientation in the everyday world, of demarcating a space for oneself. Stories provide an integrative and orienting function that is widely employed in everyday life. Knowing who one is, that is, knowing how one has become, prepares one for what or who one is to be in the future.

Autonomy involves more than momentary choice, it involves choice according to a plan. Having a plan requires a projective ability that entails a temporal attunement. Elders who suffer deficiencies or distortions in time orientation naturally appear listless and passive. Passivity sets in as agency is compromised. Agency is compromised as the ability to project a course of action into the future is affected by distortion in the underlying sense of time. Elders in whom decisional competence is intact, but lack executional ability because of physical or other incapacity (Collopy 1988: 11–12), also experience time as a gap, a hole in the world to be filled, outside their power to effectively alter. As a consequence, even elders who can make choices experience frustrations as their dependence on others creates a dissociation between the intention and the object of the action. Even though the action achieved is objectively their own, subjectively it can appear alien because the temporal continuity is interrupted. Frailties and weakness elongate the relations between intention and effect. No wonder, then, that elders exhibit hesitancy and reticence as they undertake even mundane actions because the expected outcome is temporally displaced from their habituated experience.

Agitated behavior has been defined as "inappropriate verbal, vocal, or motor activity that is not explained by needs or confusion, per se" (Cohen-Mansfield and Billig 1986: 712; also, see Cohen-Mansfield 1986). The literature on agitation primarily views these behaviors as problems of control as predicated on judgments about their social inappropriateness, but these commonly observed behaviors in institutionalized elders also seem related to distortions in the usual temporal structure of daily life in these settings. Pointing this out, of course, does not imply a causal relation between the temporal patterns of institutions and these behaviors. Other factors certainly could explain these behaviors. Whether the temporal distortions ultimately arise from physiological processes or institutional regulation, however, is not the issue, only that these are possibly meaningful behaviors that are related to environmental factors affecting time experience.

The temporal experience of elders in long-term care is profoundly affected by what I earlier termed the *fundamental anxiety*, namely, fear of death. Death cannot be far from the mind of an elder needing long-term care. In everyday life, finitude is forgotten as we projectively engage in mundane actions. Elders who need long-term care, however, frequently are unable to avoid thoughts about the meaning of life and death by immersion in daily activities. For one thing, their everyday world is radically transformed by the very need for long-term care. Barred from channeling this fundamental anxiety into meaningful daily living, elders must rely on other psychological defenses and maneuvers as they reconstitute for themselves everyday patterns and purposes. The failure of caregivers to recognize the difficulties that elders face in the everyday world of long-term care is related to their fundamental anxiety about death and seems only to compound the problem. Attention to autonomy in long-term care that focuses on maximizing choice or removing constraints seems radically misplaced since the problem of death is entirely bypassed. The very meaning and purpose of care under these circumstances need reexamination. If autonomy is a robust concept that captures actual everyday experience, then it must be made to accommodate the fundamental finite character of human existence. In long-term care, there is simply no excuse justifying avoidance of this concern.

Communication

Communication is an essential prerequisite for social action. Action in the everyday world is action in concert with others. This does not always mean that others cooperate with us in pursuing our objectives, but that even in frustrating our efforts others are communicatively engaged with us in the social world. Accordingly, not only do the changes that disability brings in one's sense of body and self deform the experience of time and space, but communicative patterns, too, are altered. Communication is often understood as a process through which information is exchanged between a sender and a receiver. In spoken language, both words and senses are exchanged, but there are also nonverbal signals that are conveyed in and through the disposition of the body. For effective communication to occur, it is necessary to have a good receiver and a good sender. Generally, human encounters in the social world are paradigmatically defined in the face-to-face relationship (Goffman 1959; 1967). What is often forgotten is that our sense of self as autonomous is socially determined in the everyday world in terms of how we are perceived by others or how we perceive that others perceive us.

Communication presumes an openness that has at least three aspects: first, the speaker must be open to modify the message to effectively communicate; second, the hearer must be able to listen (in other words, be receptive); and, third, the message must be understandable, must make sense or at least be provided with a context for further interpretation. Ironically, it seems much easier to comment on behaviors that contribute to communicative failure than to define what contributes to communicative success. For present purposes, it is sufficient to stress that one basic function of communication is to define a domain or sphere of meaning for individuals. A person's identifications then are confirmed or disconfirmed in dynamic communicative interaction.

Where communicative patterns are deformed or distorted, conflict sometimes results. When the individual is fully competent, appeal to the liberal view of autonomy as independence is at least understandable even if not always helpful. In long-term care settings, however, conflict itself is usually not the problem, but is really a symptom of a more fundamental distortion, namely, a distortion in the possibility for individuals to retain vestiges of their sense of self and personal worth. Underlying failures to communicate and achieve cooperative understanding, a process that occupies much of our everyday activity in the common social world, is sometimes a failure to express or have confirmed particular beliefs and values that comprise the stuff of our identity. The presence of unresolvable conflict is frequently a symptom of a situation in which individuals already have experienced a diminution in their sense of self-worth, rather than its cause. Such situations are important for anyone concerned about autonomy in long-term care. Indeed, the diminution of one's sense of self-worth can occur even when there is no clear evidence of conflict because the selves involved are so weakened as to be unable to engage in disputes or too disoriented to complain.

At its extreme, distortions in communication, like distortions in the individual's experience of space and time, invariably isolate individuals from participation in a shared world. This results in a corollary sense of loss in which the elder feels like a ship without an anchor, rudder, or navigation equipment. Being unable to get one's bearings or unable to change course leaves the elder in long-term care in a situation like a ship floating at the mercy of the currents and winds. No wonder, then, that sometimes erratic and seemingly irrational behavior results; just as a frightened novice sailor lost at sea might vainly attempt to take charge and steer the ship hither and yon, so too the elder manifests similar marks of anxiety and isolation. Confusion, disorientation, or wandering behavior in elders invites analysis of the communicative possibilities afforded by the caregivers and setting. Whenever communication with others is stopped, never initiated, or blocked, and access to the world is obstructed in crucial ways, not only is experience impoverished, but, more important, so is the self (Zaner 1981: 186).

In the normal everyday world there are myriad communicative patterns and styles. Communication with clerks, co-workers, friends, family, and various professionals often differ along descriptively definable lines. Indeed, one of the dominant features of the social world is the need to segregate or separate aspects of one's self as one goes about conducting one's daily affairs. This fact is important because the sense of self constituted in and through communication is dynamic. Who we are depends on where we are, what we are doing, and with whom we are engaged. Our identifications structure the repertoire of roles that we play. If these actions exhibit the marks of autonomy, then the formed identifications and patterns of behavior, the repertoire of roles, represent and express our formed sense of self. The diversity of such experiences entails that we all develop a rather wide range of typifications to be used in negotiating the world. This freedom of social action is made possible precisely by the degree to which we have formed character traits and an adequate set of habits and skills for the various encounters in the world of everyday life. Our individual sense of competence thus consists, at least in part, in the fact that we know who we are insofar as we can successfully function in a variety of circumstances.

Implications for Long-Term Care

In long-term care, some of the dominant typifications that support our communicative abilities have already broken down. For example, one deals with professionals not in discrete professional settings but as part of one's everyday private life space. Professional caregivers become intimately involved in all or most facets of one's day-to-day living, including basic activities of everyday life. Even for patients who maintain independent functioning at home or in an institutional setting, caregivers are involved in what are normally private domains, such as food preparation or have ready access to one's bedroom. This intrusion effectively means that long-term care involves degrees and kinds of intimacy with health care professionals, who are largely strangers after all, that are quite out of the ordinary in normal daily life. Given the chronic nature of caregiving relations, this intimacy challenges many of the stock concepts associated with medical ethics thinking that are based on acute care contexts.

Consider informed consent and respect for privacy. Understood in terms of the disclosure of information before a proposed diagnostic or treatment intervention, informed consent has very little relevance in long-term care (Moody 1988). First, many interactions are neither dramatic nor medical, but rather involve the provision of basic or mundane care, such as daily hygiene, feeding, and housework. Given these activities, it seems absurd to require informed consent conceived as the disclosure of information. Indeed, the legal model of informed consent as the disclosure of information simply does not fit the typical situation of long-term care. Where informed consent does seem an appropriate concern, such as in decisions to institutionalize, to increase levels of care, or to institute, withhold, or withdraw life-sustaining treatment, the situations are typically episodic and usually acute. These events punctuate long-term care much the same as acute crises punctuate normal everyday life. In long-term care, however, typical mundane encounters routinely involve matters of less pressing urgency with consequences that are less dramatic, though for that reason not less ethically important.

Second, in acute care contexts, respect for privacy is recognized as important. The paradigm seems to be that the health professional, who is generally regarded as a stranger, is allowed access to private information or examination of and performance of procedures on the patient's body only with patient consent. Intrusions into the privacy of patients is generally seen as ethically and legally problematic unless consent was secured beforehand, though there does seem to be cases in which tacit consent is sufficient. The typical realities of acute care, in which a myriad of health professionals come and go administering medications, drawing blood, performing tests, and so on—often with only some blanket general consent secured by the attending physician and not the health professionals involved directly—are conveniently ignored by the paradigm acute care model of medical ethics. Presumably because such intrusions are simply accepted as unavoidable, they have only marginal interest for and relevance to the dominant concept of autonomy as negative freedom in medical ethics. Since they typically lack the features of high risk and importance that drive the paradigm, deriving as it does from just such legal cases of conflict, these intrusions are presumably too ordinary to require explanation or analysis.

Such mundane, intrusive encounters, however, cannot be so conveniently overlooked by an ethics focusing on long-term care. (One might argue that they should not be overlooked in acute care settings either, but that point, important though it is, is tangential to the focus of this study. Indeed, one might also reasonably hope that a more adequate ethics of acute care might result from sustained reflections on the problems of long-term care, though that too lies beyond the present work.) In long-term care encounters, the typical situation becomes far more important because, in a sense, the *typical* is what structurally dominates this model of care. Typical caregiving in long-term care is less dramatic and more intimately intertwined with daily life in such a way that it is impossible to overlook questions of respect for privacy in this context.

Patterns of communication thus become important not simply in terms of disclosure of information, but in connection with the way that information is gathered, the way that behavior is observed and recorded. Institutional long-term care adopts the rituals and trappings of acute medical care, as discussed in Chapter 3, that encourage caregivers to think of elders not as individual persons, but as cases or diseases. Since the treatment is not temporally limited and since recovery and discharge from the nursing home is mostly not a real possibility, the elder is subjected to a message that only the most stalwart are able to resist for very long. Truncated communication about elders is not confined to the nursing station, but occurs daily in the halls, dayrooms, and bedrooms of elders so that soon they view each other and themselves less as unique individuals than as ideal types, as this or that kind of case, problem, or disease.

One reason why mainstream medical ethics might overlook typical encounters can be attributed to the apparent belief that the "dehumanization" and loss of actual autonomy that patients often experience in the course of hospitalization is a price worth paying for expeditious and effective treatment of acute illness. The intuition seems to be that significant losses of actual autonomy in acute care are justified by the acute, temporally limited nature of the enterprise. So the ideal of abstract autonomy as rational choice is respected in its stead. Such an intuition, however, can hardly be invoked in long-term care. Instead, long-term care routinely involves situations that can significantly affect the elder's sense of self-worth and effectively modify the elder's own self-perception. A good illustration of this point is Robert Kastenbaum's discussion of the powerful effect of statements spoken to or in the presence of geriatric patients. He gives the following examples:

> "Look at the mess you made! You'd think I didn't have anything else to do but clean up after you!"
> "This one, she can't talk. She doesn't know what you're saying."
> "She doesn't know any better. You can't tell her anything."
> "Can you do anything with this one? Boy, what a troublemaker she is!"
> "You should have seen her when she first came here, but look at her now!"
> "The poor thing would be better off going in her sleep."
> All of these comments, by the way, were completely understood by the patients even though the staff member often assumed otherwise. (1983: 6)

These statements are not just negative characterizations or descriptions; instead, they function as powerful hexes that profoundly influence the elder's self-experience which is the core of actual autonomy. As important and powerful people, those professionals charged with caring for elders were attesting to the patients' inadequacies in a fashion that was not just declaratory but also instructive or prescriptive.

These messages confirm the patients' own doubts and fears. They are instructions to be passive and ineffectual. The net effect of this kind of communication is often intensified by the reduced dimensions of the elder's world. The old person lives in an impoverished sensory and interpersonal field. Her perceptual experience is frequently monotonous, bereft of even normal stimuli and realistically achievable goals. Coupled with the elder's experiences of pain or other discomforts and the side effects of drugs, the elder experiences a profoundly altered state of consciousness; the few words spoken in her presence by "important people" can, under these circumstances, have inordinate effects. In some respects the effects might be insightfully compared with so-called hypnotic suggestions in which a person perceived as powerful makes confident judgments and demands on a person who perceives herself to be in the other's power (Kastenbaum 1983: 6).

If these observations are correct, then the contrary might also be true, namely, positive suggestion might have an equally effective response in the opposite direction. Ideally, every person in the long-term care milieu carries messages for the dependent elder. The question is whether these are messages of confidence and positive expectation or frustration and despair. Descriptions of the experience of nurses' aides (Diamond 1986; Vesperi 1983), however, do not instill hope. The cultural, economic, ethnic, and racial tensions in nursing homes are expressions of unresolved problems in the wider society. It would be unrealistic to expect that positive messages and images might be conveyed effectively to elders in long-term care without some significant improvement either in the economic and social status of the primary group of caregivers in nursing homes or structural changes in society's attitudes toward aging and the aged. Analogously, anger and frustration built up over a lifetime cannot be expected to vanish under the stressful circumstances of caring for an elder relative at home. Resentment is a powerful and pernicious attitude that infects many human relations in contemporary society (Scheler 1972). Much as one might want, it cannot be wished away by conceptual analysis. However, if positive attitudes are possible, they must be conveyed by actions, gestures, and tone of voice as well as words.

One interesting phenomenon in this regard that requires further attention is so-called baby talk to elders in long-term care. Baby talk is a simplified speech register that has special lexical items such as the use of diminutives and terms like "choo-choo" as well as morphemes, words, and constructions that are modified from adult speech. Ethnographic linguistic research suggests that baby talk is not only common but universal. It has been reported to have occurred as early as the first century B.C. and has been documented in diverse languages (Ferguson 1964; 1977). Baby talk also is truly distinctive in its paralinguistic features, especially its high pitch and its exaggerated intonation contours. Empirical research has adequately demonstrated its presence in interactions between staff members and elders in long-term care. Some see baby talk as evidence of a paternalistic or condescending attitude on the part of caregivers, whereas others point out baby talk conveys a nurturant message. As yet, there is no clear empirical evidence to decide this question. However, research on the positive or nurturant functions of baby talk is relatively undeveloped when compared with the literature on the negative, condescending, or dependency-inducing interpretation of baby talk (Caporael 1981: 876–84; Caporael et al., 1983). The implications of this work for long-term care are important.

It is natural to think that baby talk is part of the commonly reported infantilization of elders in nursing homes reported by numerous observers. For example, Kayser-Jones wrote:

> I propose that infantilization of the elderly occurs because staff who have no professional training and who are professionally unsure of themselves find it advantageous to establish a 'parent-child' relationship with the aged rather than 'adult-adult' relationship. When patients are treated like children, staff do not

have to take their life-long accomplishments into consideration, and they can more easily exercise their authority. Commands can be given and must be obeyed without question; patients do not participate in decisions about when to eat, take medications, and go to bed. Their absolute authority gives care-givers control and simplifies their work and routine. (1981: 41)

Shield reported that residents at the nursing home she observed were called by diminutive versions of their names or by generic terms, such as "honey," "dearie," "sweetie," and so on, in a section of her book titled "Old People as Children" (1988). From the context, it appears that she believed the use of such terminology is an example of infantilization. I do not know whether the baby talk actually had that function or not, but the simple use of this language should not in and of itself decide the matter. Because such behavior is regarded as failing to respect the autonomy of elders, it is concluded that elders should be communicated with in a more adult fashion. Coupled with the view of autonomy as independence, a view that assumes the elder is rational and capable of comprehension, one is lead to the conclusion that information disclosure is a primary communicative stratagem to respect elders' right of self-determination. Baby talk is clearly not information disclosure, but is seen as potentially, if not by definition, manipulative. Consideration of actual autonomy, however, seems to suggest that this conclusion might be too hasty.

If baby talk is perceived as positive and nurturing and it is not employed simply as a way to manipulate elders, then awareness of this effect would provide useful practical guidance for caregivers who are well-motivated and want to manifest positive attitudes toward elders. The demand that autonomy be respected, where autonomy is understood abstractly in terms of the idea of rational decisionmaking, could unfortunately dissuade caregivers from linguistically conveying their genuine concern. The issue of baby talk as an example of the whole domain of communicative practice in long-term care is thus of interest precisely because it underscores the fact that respecting actual autonomy entails careful attention to the concrete interactions that make up long-term care.

Some kinds of questions that might be asked with respect to particular long-term care settings are the following: First, what is the content of communication and language spoken to the dependent elder? Does it convey positive images that support and enhance the elder's sense of well-being or reflect an awareness of and respect for who the person actually is, or does it blithely disregard the identity of the dependent elder and reinforce negative attitudes that thwart actual autonomy? Second, does the environment promote or frustrate communication among elders and their normal peer-groups, between caregivers and the elder, or among professional staff or family caregivers? For example, what effect does the constant presence of the sound of a television in the day room or of frequent intercom announcements, pages for phone calls, and so on do to face-to-face communication in the nursing home? And what is gained and lost when the elder is moved from her own residence into a bustling household with children coming and going, flaunting their youth as it were? Distorted communication inevitably precludes elders from effectively expressing their autonomous identifications. Not choice as such, but the experience of self is thwarted in the worst situations. Confronted by insensitive intrusions into their fragile life space, elders are forced to adopt adaptive behavior that not surprisingly manifests itself in a confusion and disorientation, an inability to focus in conversation, and a speechless frustration.

Third, if communication occurs nonverbally as well as verbally, what messages are caregivers and elders giving to one another? Staff members who do not sit down with patients, especially patients who are bedridden or confined to wheel-chairs or geri-chairs, convey the sense that they are too busy to tarry, too preoccu-pied to be really involved with patients' needs. They tower over patients, convey-ing their authority, power, and distance.

None of these questions admits straightforward or easy answers. No algorithm exists to decipher the complex patterns of communicative action ongoing in any particular long-term care setting, much less long-term care generally. Nonetheless, insofar as communication helps establish one's place in the social world, insofar as communication is essential to establishing or maintaining a world for oneself or one's place in the world, then communication must be a central component of any reflection on the effect of long-term care on the autonomy of elders.

Finally, it is important to stress that communication in long-term care is not confined to the medical record and charts but involves a kind of oral tradition. It should not be forgotten that a good deal of emotional work is involved in long-term care: calming, cuddling, holding, and grieving. Good long-term care requires an attunement to the elder so that one knows her so intimately that one immedi-ately recognizes when she is incontinent or confused. This kind of recognition is not a matter of performing specific tasks or maintaining specialized technical skills, but involves cultivating intimate social relationships that can only be understood by reference to affectivity.

Affectivity

Persons develop and change through feeling. One important way that this occurs involves the claims that feeling places on them. Affectivity connects or separates individuals from one another. Affections literally produce changes in who we are, the most important of which help us identify with other people. The bonding of children to their parents in early childhood withstands the test of time as positive affections help forge intergenerational links. One might argue then that adult chil-dren have obligations to or at least responsibilities for their elder parents (Sommers 1987). Actual commitment to an elder, like commitment to a child, need not be reflective or deliberative, but intimately expresses the very identity of the indi-viduals involved. One is committed to a child or parent just because one is the kind of person one is; argument might persuade one about the commitments one should have, but argument makes a practical difference only if it is channeled into action. The relation to significant others is not extrinsic, but integral to the sense of one's self. This commitment is mostly prereflective, preceding and mostly pre-empting calculation of the costs of this commitment. Affectivity thus figures cen-trally in the establishment of the full range of filial responsibility (Christiansen 1983: 137–46).

Commitment to an elder parent, like a parent's commitment to his or her child, is usually forged in the continuity of time, not predicated on any particular episodes or events. Hence, one does not so much choose but finds oneself committed. This feeling explains the sense that spouses or children experience when confronted with a loved elder who needs long-term care; they are stuck without the benefit of choice. Autonomy, nonetheless, is involved insofar as that commitment can be affirmed or rejected. The apparent frequency with which individuals in our society affirm affective commitments to a frail or sick elder parent shows how strong the bonds of temporal continuity and filial responsibility actually are. That is undoubtedly why family members provide most long-term care in this country, and why nursing homes are filled mostly with elders who either lack family or whose caregiving needs exceed family capacities.

The importance of affectivity for ethics is that it is connected to traditional concepts of character, namely, distinctive dispositions that comprise the basic nature of moral personhood. It is important in this regard to distinguish an occurrent sense of autonomy, the sense that is intended when we speak of people acting autonomously in a particular circumstance or situation, and a comprehensive or dispositional sense of autonomy that defines the overall course of a person's life. Only this dispositional or comprehensive sense of autonomy allows an individual to enjoy a life that is unified, orderly, and free from self-defeating conflict over fundamental beliefs and values (Young 1986: 8). Such a dispositional sense of autonomy is possible only because the self is affectively related to itself and others. Affectivity provides the glue, as it were, that joins the various episodes and pieces of one's life into a coherent whole.

Action manifests the basic spontaneity of human life, the autonomy of persons. This manifestation, however, is not simply a matter of "gearing into" the world, of actually engaging in physical work in and on the world; rather, action also consists in various kinds of withdrawal from the everyday world of daily living. For example, one can withdraw from the ambient hustle and bustle in reverie or reading. Recollecting past memories, too, is a kind of action. To be sure, these actions have manifestations in the everyday world where they are experienced as moments of rest or islands of repose from the normal course of events, though they are hardly states of inactivity.

Daydreaming, wondering, and fantasy of various sorts including wishing or remembering involve modifications of our basic orientation to the world. These modifications in our orientation to the world provide us with the experiential depth and embellishments that persons cherish. Such activities afford the opportunity to remake the world by forming new meanings and interpretations. Indeed, this ability is tied to the very sense of an individual as a spontaneous or autonomous conscious subject and does not usually impair or conflict with an individual's ability to attend sufficiently to the practicalities of the everyday world. In effect, we manage because we are able to segregate and segment our experience into various "finite provinces of meaning" (Schutz 1971a: 207–59, 340–47). Movement from one finite province of meaning to another, especially to the finite province that Schutz termed the "paramount reality" or world of everyday experience, involves effort and the experience of shock in transitioning from the world of imagination or memory, for example, back to the world of daily life and work. Associated with these various provinces of meaning or worlds are specific feelings and moods that make these worlds hospitable or foreboding, comfortable or uncomfortable, familiar or strange (Bachelard 1969). These feelings infuse the everyday world as well by providing motivations for transitioning from one realm of meaning to another.

The death of a spouse, for example, sets a gloom on one's everyday experience as active grieving ensues. Grief involves not only feelings of loss and sadness that permeate and infuse day-to-day experiences, but requires retreat, as it were, to memory or imagination wherein the meaning of the loss and the task of reconstituting the taken-for-granted world of life is better undertaken. Similarly, illness involving pain, confusion, distraction, depression, forgetfulness, and myriad other systemic alterations in consciousness inevitably deflects the attention that the everyday world demands. Even normal and routinized activities become burdensome and difficult when illness or disability strikes. When ill, individuals necessarily retreat from the everyday world to other "worlds" or provinces of meaning. When the illness in question is systemic or chronic and the elder has already experienced a diminution of powers and abilities, the orientation to the world of everyday life, if not disengaged, is itself threatened and so the energies of the self are understandably directed away from routine activities and toward the general task of adapting or constituting new structures of meaning.

Coping strategies, in effect, involve utilizing or developing techniques to ameliorate the disengagement from the everyday world that illness or other stress foists on persons. To cope is to function in the face of adversity and suffering and the need to cope underscores not only how central the social world of everyday life is to our very existence as human persons, but the central role of feelings in the daily experience as well. One coping strategy seems to involve a positive withdrawal from the stressful world into memory or imagination; other, less adaptive forms involve confusing memory and fantasy with the actual everyday world in ways that impede the person's ability to adapt to changed circumstances. Between these extremes is a range of adaptive responses that share the common trait that feeling, not desire, reason, or will, plays the main role in constituting the meaningful connections that define the person's identity.

The world of daily life is a world of physical things including our own bodies; it is also the scene and the object of our actions. All our action in the world involves an engagement through bodily movements. Why we act, for what reason, motives, or desires is, however, related to a complex system of personal beliefs and relevances partly related to our biographical situation and partly to social typification. The typical way we act is not, as standard accounts of autonomy would have it, by rationally considering or reflecting on our desires and preferences and drawing them into accord with a hierarchy of other desires, preferences, beliefs, or values; rather, we typically feel our way through the world much like a person might feel his way through a room after all the lights have suddenly gone out. These feelings help define systems of relevance that establish meaningful expectations and interpretations of experience in the everyday world (Schutz 1970).

When I feel hunger, my stomach and body recognize it sometimes before I consciously do engaged as I am in the writing of this section. These feelings gradually rise to consciousness and interplay with other feelings that comprise a prejudgmental reflexive awareness of my place in the project at hand and that typically include links to incipient judgments about the relation of the project at hand to wider life plans. The writing as action, the hunger, and the writing as product all have their place in a system of relevance that contribute to the interpretive framework for my response. My particular response similarly reflects my habits and structured desires that are filtered in consciousness through specific kinds of feeling states: bodily feelings of sensations such as heat and cold, kinesthetic feelings of my body in action, and personal and interpersonal feelings, for example, of concern, comfort, fondness, love, pleasure, pain, or passion as well as their contraries. Action thus involves experiencing the world dynamically, as a flow of affective tonalities and textures that precede and interrelate in complex ways with cognitive understanding.

The basic affective experience that underlies the essential orientation of the agent in the world of everyday life was termed by Alfred Schutz—*fundamental anxiety* (1971a: 228). The entire system of relevances that governs us within the everyday natural attitude is founded on a formative experience of each individual, namely, I know that I shall die and I fear to die. This basic experience is the primordial anticipation from which all other experience originates. From this fundamental anxiety springs the many interrelated systems of hopes and fears, wants and satisfactions, chances and risks that incite us within the natural attitude to attempt the mastery of the world, to overcome obstacles, to draft projects, and to effortfully strive to realize them.

The fundamental anxiety itself is a corollary of our existence as human beings within the paramount reality of daily life; therefore, everyday hopes and fears and their correlated satisfactions and disappointments are grounded on and only possible within the ambient social world of everyday life. At the basis of our existence as human persons is an affective experience not of ourselves as decision makers or individuals capable of rational choice, but as finite beings. In everyday life this experience is suppressed, hidden like the framework of a house within the ceilings, floors, and walls of our projects and plans. This structure gives shape and form to the edifice as a whole; failing to attend to its significance and status is like buying a newly redecorated house that conceals serious structural flaws. The primary nature of actual autonomy cannot be adequately understood if affectivity is left unconsidered; the same attention accorded cognition and will in standard accounts of autonomy as free choice is at least required because it is not the choice or decision that defines the action so much as the felt experience of it both as my own and the embodiment of a purposive intention (Zaner 1981: 42–43).

Through kinesthetic feelings, the human person becomes present to herself and at the same time presents the self to others in the world in embodied action. Bodily action thus enacts the self in the world in a way that simultaneously reveals the self to the person and the world. That is why our experiences and our actions are always ambiguous, always uncertain both to ourselves and to others. Individuals experience themselves and the world not only through bodily feelings of mobility or immobility, but also through the experience of space and time as heavy or light, open or closed, light or dark, happy or sad, and so forth through a veritable infinity of possibilities. As affective and sentient entities, persons exist in dynamic tension with the world and others.

Persons are not neutrally situated decision makers rationally and disinterestedly calculating the costs and benefits of various alternatives. Rather, alternatives or choices impinge on them in preformed and predetermined or typified patterns, patterns that are experienced meaningfully through the vivid colors of emotion and mood and not the black and white of quantitative calculation. In a sense, the world and other persons are experienced not as nouns but adjectivally, that is, as colored by emotion and feelings, and not as the objective space-time continuum that comprises the ideal of classical physics. That is why the social world always has specific textures and colors that create eddies and cross currents in the communicative stream of everyday life. We are all able to immediately sense and speak about a room, its inhabitants, and their conversational style in terms that reflect emotional tonalities: it's a *gloomy* place; or, what a bright and lively group they are; or, what drudgery working in that office must be! Such prereflective experience is possible on the basis of the positive affective character of actual experience.

Implications for Long-Term Care

There are clinical and practical implications of these general phenomenological points. Frequently individuals who are sick for long periods of time complain about fatigue. To feel tired is obviously an accompanying symptom of certain illnesses, but fatigue as an affective quality of the experience of the world is something altogether different. Institutional fatigue, for example, is clearly identifiable: a dull, slow motor activity, shuffling walk, slow arm movements, head bowed low, stooped shoulders, a gaze devoid of usual intensity, a desire to sit almost immediately after standing or to return to bed when one is forced to leave it. The elder is much more weary than the existing conditions seem to warrant and many elders in long-term care are not even able to express the subjective character of their experience in words.

Fatigue is best understood by regarding it more as an affective, subjective experience of living through "something" rather than by examining its behavioral manifestations in isolation from the person who manifests them. The kernel of the problem is whether fatigue is best understood in terms of physiologically measurable alterations in muscle strength, which among other things can be noted by increased levels of lactic acid, or in terms of feelings occurring independently of the physiological conditions of muscle strength. Or does it have to do with both?

The character of this problem is analogous to the problem of pain, owing to a similarity in question about the role of a physiological basis in what appears to be a unique subjective experience. It may be that patients complaining about fatigue and exhibiting fatigue-related behaviors are trying to communicate by these feelings something other than what we normally construe fatigue to mean (Bergsma and Thomasma 1982: 136–37). Failure to consider this kind of alternative detracts from the question about the meaning of this experience in the context of the life plan and life story of the elder as a developed self with formed identifications. Actual autonomy is thus bypassed because the complaints of fatigue seem unrelated to choice or will except as problems or obstacles to be removed. In bypassing the affective character of fatigue, however, we bypass the concrete identity of the suffering self, a ploy that undoubtedly is reinforced by our own reticence to confront and deal with the emotional morass of our own feelings about incapacity and death.

These brief observations regarding the affective dimension of human persons and their experiences of the world bear on our understanding of the significance of autonomy for long-term care. Illness and impairment are circumstances that block one's typical or usual path or pattern of behavior in the world. In illness, whether acute or chronic, one's bodily enactment fails; hence, one's sense of personal identity is imperiled because our identity is so intimately bound up with our embodiment. Even routine action becomes effortful; engaging in activities of daily living become burdensome and wearisome. A healthy person is buoyant and free floating in the course of his or her action in the world; illness, however, weighs one down and frequently manifests itself as a lethargy or lassitude. As a result, the entire shape and texture of the world as experienced is altered for the ill person. When illness forces the elder into new living arrangements, the expected effects of illness on the elder's experience is magnified as the taken-for-granted ambient world of life, including the house or apartment, its spatial arrangement and affective tonalities, as well as its symbolic meaning, are lost and force the elder to accommodate a range of reactive feelings and emotions that engulf the self and threaten to completely erode the person's sense of identity and self-worth.

Consider the simple case of an elder who develops angina. Previously, she functioned with relative independence and self-confidence. To be sure, her actions had gradually become limited over the years, but the limitations were modest and she adapted with little difficulty. When angina occurs, the whole world is experientially transformed and placed into question in a dramatic fashion. Stairs that she was able previously to negotiate now seem to have changed their proportion; at virtually any moment the searing pain might sound off like some hidden alarm warning of limits that cannot be breached and the inescapable fact of death. New concerns become relevant, such as whether to install a lift mechanism, to move the bedroom from the second floor to the first floor turning a dining room into a bedroom and disrupting her sense of home and propriety.

The angina thus calls into question her typical and taken-for-granted experience of the world and her place therein. It presents problems in terms of relations with others, such as spouse and children, whose concern may itself threaten her fundamental sense of self-worth. It would be a mistake to argue that the issues posed here are issues of independence, though independence is certainly one of the values at stake. The concerns of relocating a bedroom to a first floor, of hiring nursing or other help or accepting the help of children are not simply questions of an abstractly autonomous individual trying to maintain independence, but affectively charged existential issues that can be meaningfully analyzed only when these features are given their proper prominence.

In circumstances like the one outlined above, it is important for caregivers to be aware that the sometimes extensive and serious modifications of life-style that become necessary in the course of long-term care force the elder to try to maintain herself in a new and different fashion. Doing so necessarily involves effort. Such effort is a signal feature of what it means to be an autonomous person or self

(Haworth 1986; Zaner 1981: 169). Accompanying this effort, no matter how feeble, maladaptive, or robust it may appear, are corollary experiences of anger, frustration, loss, and myriad emotional reactions associated with physical illness and suffering. Understanding and dealing with these reactions in a supportive fashion serve both to provide the occasion for reestablishing the connection of the ill elder with the social world and to provide the only way for caregivers to adequately understand the experienced needs of their charges.

The importance of emotional attachment in long-term care cannot be underestimated. As Timothy Diamond reported, one nursing assistant said in all seriousness that "some shit don't stink." When asked what she meant, the following reply was given: "It depends on if you like 'em and they like you, and if you know 'em pretty well; it's hard to clean somebody new, or somebody you don't like. If you like 'em, its like your baby" (1986: 1292). Similarly, the affective relationship between caregiver and elder is crucial. One cannot hold an elder as she gasps for breaths fearing that it might be the last, clean someone as you witness her own shame, or laugh with a demented or confused elder to help her maintain some modicum of social contact without affective engagement. Even routine activities, such as feeding elders, brushing their teeth, or helping them hold onto memories of the past while they try to maintain their sanity in the present, involve affective and emotional connections between caregiver and elder that are all-too-often overlooked and undervalued as the stress on service and tasks impersonalizes care to the point where bureaucratic efficiency replaces any vestige of social or ethical significance for these basic acts of care.

Summary

Phenomenologically, persons are best understood in terms of their integration in the primordial reality of the everyday world of life. This shared social world gives form and substance to the individual's actions and also provides a way to understand persons as concrete agents who exhibit complex experiential relations with the world and others. Such an orientation permits a framework for understanding autonomy that captures some of the central insights of communitarian thought, namely, the interdependent, historical, and social nature of persons, as well as the best features of agency or action-oriented theories of ethics by encouraging a concrete assessment of the meaning and function of autonomy. More important, this framework heuristically draws attention to the kind of mundane features of long-term care that ethics must accommodate.

The forgoing analysis is hardly phenomenologically complete. More can and perhaps should be said about the specific features of everyday life that I discuss as well as the many aspects that are omitted. I am also well aware that the implications for the concept of autonomy are not drawn out to the fullest extent possible. For the limited purpose of the present work, however, this analysis does provide a framework that is adequately suggestive of how a phenomenologically inspired treatment of actual autonomy in long-term care might prove ethically useful.

6

Autonomy and Long-Term Care:
Another Look

I conclude this book with a discussion that applies some elements of the theoretical framework developed earlier to a report of negotiation strategies utilized in a particular institutional setting as a way to illustrate how distortions in the social ambience of long-term care can thwart the actual autonomy of elders. The distortions affect actual autonomy not by coercion or manipulation of elders, but by modifying some of the existential conditions comprising the everyday world of experience. Autonomy, as should be patently clear, involves the way individuals live their daily lives; it is found in the nooks and crannies of everyday experience in the social world and not in the idealized paradigm of choice or decisionmaking that so dominates ethical analysis.

Social Reality of Eastside

There are myriad ways that long-term care can thwart autonomy by distorting the experience of elders. One illustration will suffice. David L. Morgan (1982) analyzed negotiation strategies surrounding the decision to move from an apartment to a nursing area in a long-term care institution; his work aptly illustrates some of the problems associated with failing to appreciate the concrete reality of elders as persons. Morgan regards the move to the nursing area as a key "benchmark" and discusses the negotiations that surrounded the move as falling into a sequence of five strategies that residents are likely to employ. First, they attempt to disguise their health problems; second, they minimize the problems that cannot be disguised; third, they deny that their problem requires treatment or that the nursing area is the appropriate locus for treatment; fourth, they seek alternatives to a move to the nursing area; and finally, they create conflict among the home's staff. Although these stages summarize a general path of negotiations, not every resident passes through each stage and movement back and forth between stages is not uncommon (Morgan 1982: 43).

Morgan primarily discusses how staff members respond to each of these tactics, but initially provides a characterization of the social setting that staff and residents helped to create. For example, the head nurse regularly denied that anyone in the apartment area was really well and that each was at least a little confused. She and the other staff members engaged in a continual process of monitoring the residents in order to see who was having trouble. Importantly, these informal reviews attached medical significance to signals such as mobility limitations, general instability, drooling, occasional mild confusion (e.g., losing track of time), and temporary limitations in routine activities (e.g., not appearing well-dressed at meals). Interestingly, this monitoring seemed to be the main interactional goal of staff. Not surprisingly, residents were quite aware of this monitoring of their daily lives and undertook attempts to evade monitoring as their first line of defense against a move to the nursing area. The general picture of the social world of Eastside that emerges in Morgan's description is one involving tension and an adversarial atmosphere in which residents typically became preoccupied with avoiding becoming trapped in the sick role.

Although Morgan did not discuss the point, it seems clear that staff both adopted and attempted to enforce the expectations associated with the sick role. As described by Talcott Parsons, this role has four essential features: first, recovery from the incapacity is seen as being beyond the power of the person's will; second, the incapacity is seen as a legitimate basis for exemption from normal role and task responsibilities; in a sense the individual is not held responsible and is expected to surrender normal role responsibilities; third, the sick role is legitimated as a special social role because the condition is both undesirable and entails the obligation that the person do everything necessary to get well; and fourth, since the natural course of events cannot be relied on to improve the condition, the sick person is responsible to seek out competent professional help (Parsons 1951: 428–79; 1958). As discussed in Chapter 3, the sick role concept supports professional over patient autonomy and assumes an acute concept of illness. The apparent inappropriateness of this model for the elders at Eastside seems to underlie much of the tension that Morgan observed.

The first and most common way that residents disguised health problems was through appearance, that is, by trying to appear competent and capable in public. This disguise was accomplished by displaying good appearance when expected, for example, at mealtimes. Indeed, it was not uncommon for residents to prepare for particularly demanding public performances by resting prior to the activity. Such behavior, which might otherwise be described simply as prudent or practical, was itself noticed by staff and, indeed, other residents as grounds for more careful monitoring. Rather than supporting adaptation to illness, both staff and other residents upheld an apparently unrealistic ideal of independence. Unsuccessful attempts to disguise accidents and other critical incidents arising from failing health led to bargaining precisely when the resident was least able to cope. At the point when they were most vulnerable, residents were subjected to the assumption that they could truly negotiate and bargain rather than offered a supportive, nurturing style of interaction.

Morgan reports that the medical staff had warned one woman that her general instability made a disabling fall probable if she continued living in her apartment. Having slipped on a bathroom scale and cut her leg, she attempted to care for herself rather than to admit to the fall. The wound ulcerated and she was unable to leave her bed. At this point her absences from the dining room were noted and she was immediately moved to the nursing area where she remained bedridden for two months due as much to mental collapse as to the condition of her leg (1982: 43–44). In effect, staff actively strove to discover incapacities on the part of residents and residents strove to avoid the consequence of such discovery, namely, a forced negotiation regarding a move to the nursing home; the conflict that resulted from each side's efforts to control the unacceptable behavior of the other produced still higher levels of the undesired behavior. Morgan points out that most of the so-called negotiations at Eastside tended to heighten rather than to resolve conflict. It is important to understand both why this was so and how incorporating a phenomenologically accurate view of actual autonomy is helpful.

Appeal to Autonomy as Independence

It is important to note, however, that on a superficial reading the traditional view of autonomy seems to be recommended by just such a case as this. One might easily argue that the staff at Eastside were guilty of obsessive interference in the lives of the residents which resulted in their engendering paranoia regarding the move to the nursing area. In a sense, the staff seemed bent on constant interference and involvement in the lives of the residents. It created a conflictual situation in which interactions between residents and staff were structured by suspicion and distrust. Due to the disproportionate power of staff over residents, appeals to the autonomy of the residents, for example, as expressed by the residents' rights to be left alone or to decide regarding the style and timing of care, serve to protect elders in situations in which they are most decisionally vulnerable. That observation is true enough but it only scratches the surface of the social world of Eastside and hardly helps us think creatively about enhancing the autonomy of institutionalized elders generally. The traditional concept of autonomy simply does not help address what is most ethically problematic about this situation nor suggest ways how the deficiencies might be remedied. An alternative analysis is required.

A Phenomenologically Informed Analysis

The phenomenological view of the social nature of persons articulated in Chapter 5 provides an alternative framework for interpreting the situation at Eastside. Importantly, this framework focuses attention not on the standard concepts of patients' rights and the value of autonomy as independence, but rather invites critical reflection on the structure of everyday life at Eastside. In the interest of fairness and conciseness this analysis is confined to descriptions and observations provided in Morgan's own account in order to prevent an imaginative, but possibly inaccurate, interpretation that simply reads in concerns that are empirically unfounded. This analysis underscores an important methodological point about the phenomenological framework developed earlier, namely, that it requires attention to the actual empirical detail in situations of long-term care. The primary implication of this framework is less to draw general normative conclusions than to offer a practically defensible and useful ethical analysis that is anchored in accurate descriptive assessment.

At Eastside, the expectations of elders were in various degrees and manners influenced by the monitoring actions of staff. Apparently, these monitoring activities produced just the opposite of the intended effect. Instead of bringing health problems to the attention of staff to allow for efficient and expeditious treatment, the adversarial style of interaction between staff and residents encouraged residents to develop specific strategies to minimize their health problems. Morgan noted that two such strategies were evident: the routinization of daily activities and the enlistment of social support. Each of these strategies viewed in its own terms constitutes a reasonable coping strategy for individuals experiencing diminished physical capacity. In the interpretive frame of Eastside, however, these actions were taken by staff as *prima facie* evidence of diminished capacity constituting grounds for moving a resident into the nursing area in order to forestall more serious consequences. The dominance of these beneficent intentions on the part of staff precluded or preempted other alternatives. Concern for the physical well-being of residents at the price of ignoring their valiant, if sometimes vain, attempts to maintain integrity of self and minimal social functioning had deleterious consequences on the entire social fabric of the institution.

Morgan reported that residents regarded enlisting social support from other residents as a potential resource, whereas in reality active peer support for health-related problems was relatively uncommon. Morgan explained that this was due to resistance against "being dragged down," namely, the belief that it was wrong to sacrifice one's own health by caring for others, the exception being caring for one's spouse (1982: 44). As a result, residents seemed to experience unbearable isolation at the very time that they experienced fundamental threats to their sense of self. Staff accused residents who relied on relatives or other residents for support as placing unreasonable burdens on others who were no more competent than they themselves: "They argued that the health of the potential source of support was in fact no more certain than the health of the intended recipient. They told residents that their use of another person as a source of support was dangerous to them *and* to their friend" (Morgan 1982: 45)

In effect, the ability of residents to recognize their own limitations and to autonomously ask for and accept help, an otherwise positive sign of mature judgment, was made a problem at Eastside. The effect was a further erosion of the social fabric that supported elders' sense of self-worth. Whether this contributed to or was an outcome of the social setting is hard to say, but it existed correlative to a group norm that supported the communal desire that the home be filled with largely outwardly healthy and competent members. It was clearly exercised at the expense of declining individuals and the few individuals who were willing to risk the censure of the medical staff and the gossip of their fellow residents to supportively respond to another elder's need.

Applying these observations to the social world at Eastside leads to the conclusion that what Morgan describes is a world composed of individuals who manifest counterdependence, the aversion for dependence of all sorts; this conclusion reinforces the liberal view of autonomy, namely, that of persons as isolated, egoistic individuals. Denial is an important psychological defense mechanism that seemed to function socially as well in the way that negotiation was conducted at Eastside. For example, when the focus shifted toward the implications of a particular resident's problem that could not be effectively disguised or minimized, residents attempted to remove or deny the staff's version of the facts. In disguising and minimizing the problem, residents attempted to reject the need for negotiation regarding movement to the nursing area. A corollary strategy was to deny the staff's assessment of the problem. Clearly, staff possessed superior medical knowledge, but that knowledge was not persuasive with residents who compared themselves with other residents who were more ill. Residents would commonly say, "I am not as bad off as so and so." Another tactic was to dispute the consequences of the move. They argued, probably correctly, that a move to the nursing area would make them depressed or anxious. Also, residents seemed to believe that life in the nursing area was unbearable.

By denying the benefits of treatment, residents directly attacked the rationale behind the attempt to move them, namely, that a move was for their own good, and focused instead on psychological issues such as depression or agitation that are sufficiently ambiguous that even staff had to acknowledge them (Morgan 1982: 45). One "trump" move that staff had available was to shift the burden of proof from their having to justify moving a resident to the nursing area to the resident's need to provide evidence of competence. Although some residents considered leaving the home as a countermove, this alternative was seldom exercised. Staff tried to convince residents of the lack of alternatives by offering them temporary, short-term stays in the nursing area, but Morgan pointed out that staff did admit to bargaining in bad faith by claiming to offer a solution to a temporary problem when what they actually intended was to demonstrate a real lack of alternatives to a move to the nursing area (1982: 46).

Ironically, the possibility of temporary stays in the nursing area was reported to be one of Eastside's special advantages for newly arrived residents. However, these residents quickly learned that once in the nursing area it became easier for staff to keep them there permanently. For this reason, patients sometimes sought other alternatives such as trying to gain admission to hospitals when acute care was necessary despite the additional cost. Morgan raises the relevant question why more medical care was not provided outside the nursing area since that space in the facility carried such negative associations for the elders. A correlative question is how did elders perceive life in the nursing area that they were willing to forgo needed care rather than endure the transfer.

Since the alternative at Eastside was a transfer to the nursing area or nothing, the situation was clearly a no-win one for the elders. The only real alternative for residents as they experienced inevitable deterioration was movement to the nursing area. No effort was made to understand the elders' as unique individuals. The only positive sense of self in evidence was tied up with the rather abstract concept of independent functioning; reciprocal or mutual exchanges or interchanges never seemed to develop. In this sense, there were no community supports to sustain elders through the emotional strain of the move. Without independence, they were nothing, but with it they proudly lived in affective isolation from one another.

The nursing area represented a loss of their generalized social self. It represented isolation and falling under the authoritarian control of staff who seemed preoccupied with physical considerations and little with psychosocial and interpersonal concerns. Indeed, Morgan pointed out that a tradeoff between health-related benefits and social costs is a general feature of transitions along the health care continuum for elders (1982: 47). The question is whether such tradeoffs and resultant costs to patient autonomy really are inevitable or do they represent a systemic failure at Eastside to appreciate the tenuous nature of human personhood and personal worth?

What seems peculiar about Eastside is the way that the transition between apartment living and existence in the nursing area constituted less a transition than a shock, a shattering shift into a different multiple reality, one that cost the individual a sense of personal identity and social functioning. In a way, the nursing area represented a loss of the paramount reality because patients therein could not function as true social agents. It seems that residents believed that once in the nursing area, they would be literally at the end of their rope without prospect of further meaningful interaction; most troubling is the apparent fact that apartment life did not seem to afford much in the way of a rich social existence either. Was the staff guilty of coercing patients into abject dependence? Certainly some residents moved into the nursing area as a result of serious illness and not because of the preferences or overprotective concern of staff members. Nevertheless, the way that the staff typified residents as patients, even when they lived in their own apartments, by assuming that they needed care and were neither able to make decisions for themselves nor able to function in any way that preserved their sense of dignity, created the impression that the nursing area symbolized the profound loss of autonomy that, perhaps more important, permeated everyday life at Eastside. Since the staff seemed quite incapable of providing patients with any sense of hope or meaningful interactions, they were hardly perceived as nurturing, but profoundly threatening to the elder's sense of self. Inevitably, conflict resulted but the conflict was the tip of the proverbial iceberg. The real ethical problems at Eastside were far deeper and more significant.

Morgan points out that conflict did work as a tactic for delaying moves, but it was a last ditch strategy. Putting up a fight cost residents the sympathy and support of their peers and led to social isolation even when they retained their own apartments. Conflict took two forms: either eliciting outside support, such as family and members of Eastside's board of trustees, or the home's top administrator. The fact that conflict was always a possibility points to an important caveat in using the term *negotiation* to describe staff and elder interactions in this setting. Each side viewed its objectives as nonnegotiable, and so there was little or nothing that would bring either side closer to the other's point of view. As a consequence, the process of "negotiation" was a bad faith effort from the start. It was a no-win situation for all parties and contributed to the frustration on both sides. What underlies the difference between these two perspectives? Morgan argued that the basic conflict involved the staff's attempt to prevent the "premature" death of elders whereas the elders seemed intent to avoid a life-style that amounted to "social" death (1982: 48).

Lessons from Eastside

It must be stressed that my discussion of Morgan's description of Eastside involves reading "between the lines" of both the report and its analysis. Such reading is precisely what is required if we are to take seriously the phenomenological account of autonomy developed earlier. Simply focusing on obvious instances of autonomous behavior or their frustration, such as those comfortably expressed in terms of patient's rights and decisional conflict, is inadequate. Eastside presents a case in which the social structure itself did not seem conducive to supporting the full range of human autonomy and respect for persons, with the failures noted by Morgan representing a surface analysis. Eastside seems to present a striking instance in which the possibly beneficent concern of staff led to resident loneliness by precisely stimulating elders' isolation from those around them. Loneliness can be understood either as social isolation or emotional isolation (Mullins and McNicholas 1986).

Loneliness as social isolation results from losses in the individual's support system, decreased participation in social activities, and a reduced sense of social and personal fulfillment (Mullins and McNicholas 1986). Importantly, absence of social reinforcements has been shown to induce loneliness. Emotional isolation involves discrepancy between the individual's own sense of self-identity, the vision of her ideal self, and the image of herself reflected in how others see her. Features of this loneliness involve feelings of loss, distress, or separation and isolation. The essential component is the affective element, namely, the feeling or emotion that attaches to the subjective experience of being alone. In this context loneliness involves a psychological and behavioral response to the condition of actual or perceived social isolation. Thus, loneliness can be viewed as an affective experience in which an elder experiences being apart from others and apart from familiar support systems and personally meaningful possessions.

This experience of loneliness can lead to or include the realization that social contacts are diminishing, lacking, or are not qualitatively satisfactory (Mullins and McNicholas 1986: 58). Loneliness, however, is not directly able to be correlated with the amount of social contacts as such. Living alone, for example, does not necessarily result in an individual feeling lonely. In the case of Eastside, communal living seemed to stimulate a sense or fear of loneliness that would occur as the result of being transferred from the residence to the nursing area, but loneliness was actually built into the everyday patterns of interaction in which unrealistic and ideal independence was fostered as a social ideal. Hence, an important ethical question here concerns not only the inability or unwillingness of staff to assess this phenomenon, but their failure to address the underlying typified perceptions of the nursing area on the elders' sense of identity.

These observations on Morgan's description of negotiation strategies at Eastside illustrate both the ethical complexity associated with a view of autonomy that is concretely grounded in an understanding of the social nature of persons and how limited an orientation is that focuses on decisionmaking and conflict. Of course the true reality of Eastside cannot be assessed from an armchair. The theory of autonomy developed earlier requires a *concrete* understanding of elders in long-term care. Discussion of Eastside is employed only as a convenient, but admittedly limited, illustration.

Conclusion

Ethics must deal with problems not simply of *doing* good or *producing* good, but of *being* good. It must expand its usual concerns beyond dilemmas, problems, or quandaries to address questions of character and virtue. Contemporary ethics tends to miss the connection between the rites and routines of everyday life and moral action because it focuses on moral binds and quandaries, namely, special situations in which we do not know what to do. Emphasis is placed on situations and circumstances in which the individual is thrown outside of routine ways of acting, is confronted with choices, and so is puzzled about what to so. In such kinds of cases the individual appears to be poised between clear alternatives, uncertain as to which way to proceed. Too little attention is devoted to those great overarching rhythms and patterns that make up everyday life. If autonomy is to be a significant concept for long-term care, then these interstitial features and patterns need to be examined. For ethics to helpfully reflect on life as it actually is lived, attention to routine and habitual behaviors and actions must be fostered (May 1986: 56).

In the foregoing discussion, I argued that the concept of autonomy properly understood requires that individuals be seen in essential interrelationship with others and the world. This view was developed in a general way in terms of a discussion of the social world of everyday life and the temporal, spatial, communicative, and affective dimensions of personhood and in terms of a view that actual autonomy of persons fundamentally involves who the individual is and how she has developed as a formed self. In exploring the meaning and function of autonomy and long-term care, I have argued that autonomy is important both normatively and conceptually in ethics and long-term care. The position defended does not preclude the possibility that other concepts are also important and fundamental. The astute reader will have seen, for example, that I am committed to the importance of beneficence in long-term care. I do not, however, try to assimilate the concept of beneficence or other values with that of autonomy, nor do I fully analyze the nature of the relationship between these values and concepts to the extent likely to satisfy every reader. Only when it seemed appropriate or necessary for the flow of my argument did I suggest how particular points might be approached.

Throughout this study an expansive use of the liberal concept of autonomy as independence and noninterference was opposed on the grounds that it is really a limited political/legal concept that is woefully incomplete for the full purposes of ethical theory. Its most notable deficiency is its failure to accommodate a concrete understanding of persons and the nature of ethical responsibilities in the

everyday world. In various guises the liberal view of autonomy influences thinking about long-term care. For example, social perceptions that autonomy means
independence leads to the attitude of counterdependence in which elders feel obligated to avoid anything that appears to involve dependence; society for its part
supports this behavior by institutional arrangements that assure that the full price
of independence is paid. The lack of adequate long-term care insurance, including
home care services and support in this country, often makes illness or disability
for elders an all or nothing choice: either one accepts full dependence in a hospital or nursing home because medical problems are not attended to in a timely fashion, or one struggles with the functional disabilities associated with the illnesses
of being old without adequate care until disaster arrives. Positively, elders do enjoy
important and significant benefits afforded by a panoply of rights that is supported
by the liberal ideals of noninterference and independence.

Long-term care is required precisely because elders experience to some degree
a practical loss of functional abilities that we routinely associate with autonomy.
They lose various abilities to act in the world and so require more than the usual
amounts and kinds of support and care from others. The ambivalence of our society toward the old and long-term care is illustrated in the fact that we seem to
want both to support the right of frail elders to deny their need for care—in short,
we support their right to noninterference regardless of the great personal cost—
and yet we recognize that those who cannot care for themselves and who place
undue burdens on family members require specialized professional care. Institutional care, particularly skilled-level nursing care, thus represents the extreme alternative: a situation in which autonomy gives way to sometimes abject dependence.
Consistent with our society's concern for independence, however, is the development of efforts to secure institutionalized elders' rights to noninterference by even
benevolently motivated health care professionals. Unfortunately, this either/or situation does not conceptually capture the mundane ethical reality of either autonomy
or long-term care, a reality that exists somewhere between the ideal of individuals
as isolated, rational decision makers and individuals as passively dependent.

Autonomy as negative freedom or liberty focuses on how individuals want to
act, what they want to do. This focus, however, ignores or fails to take into consideration the capacity of individuals to reflect on and adopt particular attitudes
toward their desires and values. It also ignores how their desires and preferences
were acquired; as a result, a rather abstract view of persons results. However, if it
matters ethically to persons not only that they have particular values or beliefs,
but that they have acquired these values and beliefs in certain ways, then an account that incorporates developmental aspects of human individuals is necessary.
Gerald Dworkin argued that what is necessary is a "fuller appreciation of their
higher-order preferences" (1988: 106), but this in itself is too general a point. It
implies a view of the person that is largely a philosophical fiction, an individual
capable of clear self-conscious, critical reflective ability.

In this regard, Dworkin's recent work on autonomy (1988) seems to want it
both ways, namely, to retain talk of second-order preferences and the critical and
reflective abilities necessary to estimate them, yet recognize that autonomy in the
everyday sense cannot meet this philosophical ideal. The issue here is extremely

important. While I have broached this issue mainly by indirection, favoring a developmental approach that at the same time acknowledges the importance of identifications, my view of identification is one that does not require explicit critical self-reflection. Instead, I have suggested a process that ranges from such an idea all the way to the opposite extreme of testing and modifying of beliefs and values in everyday practical action and experience. Critics admittedly might claim that so wide a view verges on making autonomy so all-encompassing as to be vacuous. I do not think that is necessarily the case, but I admit that I have not conclusively proved the point here. Since my concern is the relevance of autonomy to long-term care, however, this omission seems defensible.

Elders needing long-term care, after all, suffer not only from physical impairments and incapacities, but cognitive and memory deficits as well. Confusion and wandering are prominent behaviors of institutionalized elders. If the concept of autonomy is to have any ethically significant applicability to this population, then it will need to have more elasticity than is usually evident in standard philosophical treatments. We are going to have to recognize autonomy in rather mundane and ordinary settings and circumstances that philosophical analysis has largely left unexplored. Characterizing autonomy in this rather broad way, to repeat, is not equivalent to claiming that the analysis is complete, but only that the course has been correctly charted. Although concern for theoretical completeness is philosophically compelling, it may not be ethically crucial if the account of autonomy proffered affords a framework for practically rethinking the ethics of long-term care. For present purposes, I am happy to sacrifice theoretical completeness for practical efficacy.

Bibliography

Adler, Jonathan E. 1987. "Moral Development And the Personal Point of View." In Eva Feder Kittay and Diana T. Meyers (eds.), *Woman and Moral Theory*. Totowa, NJ: Rowan & Littlefield, 205–34.

Agich, George J. 1981. "The Question of Technology in Medicine." In Stephen Skousgaard (ed.), *Phenomenology and Understanding Human Destiny*. Washington, DC: Center for Advanced Research in Phenomenology and University Press of America, 81–92.

———. 1982. "The Concept of Responsibility in Medicine." In George J. Agich (ed.), *Responsibility in Health Care*. Dordrecht, Holland: D. Reidel, 53–73.

———. 1983a. "Disease and Value: A Rejection of the Value Neutrality Thesis." *Theoretical Medicine* 4: 27–41.

———. 1983b. "Scope of the Therapeutic Relationship." In Earl E. Shelp (ed.), *The Clinical Encounter*. Dordrecht, Holland: D. Reidel, 233–50.

———. 1986. "Economic Cost and Moral Value." In George J. Agich and Charles E. Begley (eds.), *The Price of Health*. Dordrecht, Holland: D. Reidel, 23–42.

———. 1987. "Incentives and Obligations under Prospective Payment." *Journal of Medicine and Philosophy* 11: 123–44.

———. 1990a. "Medicine as Business and Profession." *Theoretical Medicine* 11: 311–24.

———. 1990b. "Rationing and Professional Autonomy." *Law, Medicine & Health Care* 18 (Spring–Summer): 77–84.

———. 1990c. "Reassessing Autonomy in Long-Term Care." *Hastings Center Report* 20 (6): 12–17.

———. 1991. "Access to Health Care: Charity and Rights." In Thomas J. Bole and William B. Bondeson (eds.), *Rights to Health Care*. Dordrecht, Holland: Kluwer, 185–98.

Altman, Irwin. 1975. *The Environment and Social Behavior: Privacy, Personal Space, Territory, Crowding*. Monterey, CA: Brooks/Cole.

Ambrogi, Donna M. 1990. "Nursing Home Admissions: Problematic Process and Agreements." *Generations* 14 (Supplement): 72–74.

Ambrogi, Donna M., and L. E. Gerard. 1986. *Autonomy of Nursing Home Residents: A Study of California Nursing Home Admission Agreements*. San Francisco, CA: Law Center on Long Term Care.

Ambrogi, Donna M., and Frances Leonard. 1988a. "The Impact of Nursing Home Admission Agreements on Resident Autonomy." *Gerontologist* 28 (Supplement, June): 82–89.

————. 1988b. *Nursing Home Admission Agreements: State Studies, National Recommen-dations.* San Francisco, CA: California Law Center on Long Term Care.

American College of Physicians. 1984a. "American College of Physicians Ethics Manual. Part I." *Annals of Internal Medicine* 101 (1): 129–37.

————. 1984b. "American College of Physicians Ethics Manual. Part II." *Annals of Internal Medicine* 101 (2): 263–74.

Appelbaum, Paul S., and Thomas G. Gutheil. 1979. "Rotting with Their Rights On: Constitution Theory and Reality in Drug Refusal by Psychiatric Patients." *Bulletin of the American Journal of Psychiatry in the Law* 7: 308–17.

Azarnoff, R. S., and A. E. Scharach. 1988. "Can Employees Carry the Eldercare Burden?" *Personnel Journal* (September): 60–65.

Bachelard, Gaston. 1969. *The Poetics of Space.* Maria Jolas (tr.), Boston: Beacon Press.

Baier, Annette. 1985. *Postures of the Mind: Essays on Mind and Morals.* Minneapolis: University of Minnesota Press.

Baum, W. 1980–81. "The Therapeutic Value of Oral History." *International Journal of Aging and Human Development* 12 (1): 49–53.

Beauchamp, Tom L., and James F. Childress. 1983. *Principles of Biomedical Ethics*, Third Edition. New York and Oxford: Oxford University Press.

Beauvoir, Simone de. 1972. *The Coming of Age.* Patrick O'Brien (tr.), New York, Putnam.

Bellah, Robert N., Richard Madsen, William N. Sullivan, Ann Swindler, and Steven M. Tipton. 1985. *Habits of the Heart: Individualism and Commitment in American Life.* Berkeley, CA: University of California Press.

Belson, B. S., *et al.* 1988. "Meeting Employees' Needs For Elder Care." *Compensation and Benefits Management* 4 (2): 117–21.

Benhabib, Seyla. 1987. "The Generalized and the Concrete Other: The Kohlberg–Gilligan Controversy and Moral Theory." In Eva Feder Kittay and Diana T. Meyers (eds.), *Women and Moral Theory.* Totowa, NJ: Rowan & Littlefield, 154–77.

Benjamin, Martin, and Joy Curtis. 1981. *Ethics in Nursing.* New York: Oxford University Press.

Benn, S. I. 1976. "Freedom, Autonomy and the Concept of a Person." *Proceedings of The Aristotelian Society* 76: 109–30.

Bergmann, Frithjof. 1977. *On Being Free.* Notre Dame, IN: University of Notre Dame Press.

Bergsma, Jurrit, and David Thomasma. 1982. *Health Care: Its Psychosocial Dimensions.* Pittsburgh, PA: Duquesne University Press.

Berlin, Isaiah. 1969. *Four Essays on Liberty.* Oxford: Oxford University Press.

Bettelheim, Bruno. 1960. *The Informed Heart: Autonomy in a Mass Society.* New York: Free Press.

Bishop, Christine E., and Sarita L. Karon. 1989. "The Composition of Home Health Care Expenditure Growth." *Home Health Care Services Quarterly* 10 (1/2): 139–75.

Bittner, Egon. 1973. "Objectivity and Realism in Sociology." In George Psathas (ed.), *Phenomenological Sociology.* New York: Wiley, 109–25.

Blakeslee, Jill, Beyrl Goldman, and Dawn Papougenis. 1990. "Untying the Elderly: Kendal's Restraint-Free Program at Longwood and Crosslands." *Generations* 14 (Supplement): 79–80.

Bogan, James, and Daniel Farrell. 1978. "Freedom and Happiness in Mill's Defense of Liberty." *Philosophical Quarterly* 28: 325–38.

Booth, Tim. 1986. "Institutional Regimes and Induced Dependency in Homes for the Aged." *Gerontologist* 26(4): 418–23.

Bosch, Gerhard. 1970. *Infantile Autism: A Clinical and Phenomenological–Anthropological Investigation Taking Language as the Guide*. Derek and Inge Jordan (trs.), Berlin/Heidelberg/New York: Springer-Verlag.

Bowlby, John. 1969. *Attachment and Loss: Volume I, Attachment*. New York: Basic Books.

———. 1973. *Attachment and Loss: Volume II, Separation*. New York: Basic Books.

———. 1980. *Attachment and Loss: Volume III, Loss*. New York: Basic Books.

Brent, Ruth Stumpe. 1984. "Advocacy Designed in the Nursing Home: Cultivating Public And Private Spaces for the Newly Admitted Resident." In Stuart F. Spicker and Stanley R. Ingman (eds.), *Vitalizing Long-Term Care: The Teaching Nursing Home and Other Perspectives*. New York: Springer, 159–76.

Brock, Dan W. 1988. "Paternalism and Autonomy." *Ethics* 98: 550–65.

Brody, Elaine M. 1985. "Parent Care as Normative Family Stress." *Gerontologist* 25(1): 19–29.

Brown, Robert N. 1985. "Contract Rights to Admission, Transfer and Discharge." *American Health Care Association Journal* 11(3): 17–19.

Buchanan, Allen E. 1981. "Medical Paternalism." In Marshall Cohen, Thomas Nagel, and Thomas Scanlon (eds.), *Medicine and Moral Philosophy*. Princeton, NJ: Princeton University Press, 214–34.

———. 1983. "The Limits of Proxy Decision-Making." In Rolf Sartorius (ed.), *Paternalism*. Minneapolis: University of Minnesota Press, 153–70.

———. 1991. "Rights, Obligations, and the Special Importance of Health Care." In Thomas J. Bole and William B. Bondeson (eds.), *Rights to Health Care*. Dordrecht, Holland: Kluwer, 169–84.

Buchanan, Allen E., and Dan W. Brock. 1989. *Deciding For Others: The Ethics of Surrogate Decision Making*. Cambridge: Cambridge University Press.

Buckingham, C. 1987. *Admission Agreements of Maryland Nursing Homes*. Baltimore: Maryland Department of Health and Mental Hygiene.

Burrow, Jay A. 1988. *The Ages of Man*. Oxford: Oxford University Press.

Butler, L. W., and Paul W. Newacheck. 1981. "Health and Social Factors Relevant to Long-Term-Care Policy." In Judith Meltzer, Frank Farrow, and Harold Richman (eds.), *Policy Options in Long-Term Care*. Chicago: University of Chicago Press, 38–77.

Butler, Robert. 1963. "The Life Review: An Interpretation of Reminiscence in the Aged." *Psychiatry* 26 (February): 65–76.

———. 1974. "Successful Aging and the Role of the Life Review." *Journal of The American Geriatrics Society* 22 (12): 529–35.

———. 1975. *Why Survive? Being Old in America*. New York: Harper and Row.

———. 1980–81. "The Life Review: An Unrecognized Bonanza." *International Journal of Aging and Human Development* 12 (1): 35–38.

Callahan, Daniel. 1984. "Autonomy: A Moral Good Not a Moral Obsession." *Hastings Center Report* 14 (5): 40–42.

———. 1985. "What Do Children Owe Their Elderly Parents?" *Hasting Center Report* 15 (2): 32–33.

———. 1987. *Setting Limits: Medical Goals in an Aging Society*. New York: Simon and Schuster.

Caplan, Arthur L. 1984. "Is Aging a Disease?" In Stuart F. Spicker and Stanley R. Ingman (eds.), *Vitalizing Long-Term Care: The Teaching Nursing Home and Other Perspectives*. New York: Springer, 14–28.

Caplan, Arthur, H. Tristram Engelhardt, Jr., and Joseph McCartney, eds. 1981. *Concepts of Disease: Interdisciplinary Perspectives*. Reading, MA: Addison-Wesley.

Caporael, Linnda R. 1981. "The Paralanguage of Caregiving: Baby Talk to the Institutionalized Aged." *Personality and Social Psychology* 40: 876–84.

Caporael, Linnda R., Marlene P. Lukaszewski, and Glen H. Culbertson. 1983. "Secondary
Baby Talk: Judgments by Institutionalized Elderly and Their Caregivers." *Journal
of Personality and Social Psychology* 44: 746–54.

Childress, James F. 1982. *Who Should Decide? Paternalism in Health Care.* New York
and Oxford: Oxford University Press.

———. 1990. "The Place of Autonomy in Bioethics." *Hastings Center Report* 20 (1): 12–
17.

Christiansen, Andrew J. 1983. *Autonomy and Dependence in Old Age: An Ethical Analysis.* Yale University Doctoral Dissertation. Ann Arbor: University Microfilms.

Christiansen, Drew. 1978. "Dignity in Aging—Notes on Geriatric Ethics." *Journal of
Humanistic Psychology* 18 (2): 41–54.

Christie, Ronald J., and C. Barry Hoffmaster. 1986. *Ethical Issues in Family Medicine.*
New York: Oxford University Press.

Christman, John. 1988. "Constructing the Inner Citadel: Recent Work on the Concept of
Autonomy." *Ethics* 99 (October): 109–24.

———. ed. 1989. *The Inner Citadel: Essays on Individual Autonomy.* New York and Oxford:
Oxford University Press.

Clark, Margaret. 1971. "Cultural Values and Dependency in Later Life." In Donald O.
Cowgill and Lowell D. Holmes (eds.), *Aging and Modernization.* New York:
Appelton-Century-Crofts, 263–74.

Cluff, Leighton E. 1981. "Chronic Disease, Function and the Quality of Care." *Journal of
Chronic Disease* 34: 299–304.

Code of Federal Regulations: Public Health. Title 42, Part 405, Subpart K. Conditions of
Participation: Skilled Nursing Facilities. Office of The Federal Register, National
Archives and Records Administration. Washington, DC: U.S. Government Printing
Office, October 1, 1987a.

Code of Federal Regulations: Public Health. Title 42, Part 405, Subpart S. Certification
Procedures For Providers and Suppliers of Services. Office of The Federal Register, National Archives and Records Administration. Washington, DC: U.S. Government Printing Office, October 1, 1987b.

Code of Federal Regulations: Public Health. Title 42, Part 442, Subparts D and E. Skilled
Nursing Requirements and Intermediate Care Facility Requirements: All Facilities.
Office of The Federal Register, National Archives and Records Administration.
Washington, DC: U.S. Government Printing Office, October 1, 1987c.

Cohen, Elias S. 1985. "Autonomy and Paternalism: Two Goals in Conflict." *Law, Medicine and Health Care* 13 (4): 145–50.

———. 1988. "The Elderly Mystique: Constraints on the Autonomy of the Elderly With
Disabilities." *Gerontologist* 28 (Supplement, June): 24–31.

Cohen, Uriel, and Gerald D. Weisman. 1990. "Environmental Design to Maximize
Autonomy for Older Adults with Cognitive Impairments." *Generations* 14 (Supplement): 75-78.

———. 1991. *Holding Onto Home: Designing Environments for People With Dementia.*
Baltimore: Johns Hopkins University Press.

Cohen-Mansfield, Jiska, and Nathan Billig. 1986. "Agitated Behaviors in The Elderly I. A
Conceptual Review." *Journal of the American Geriatrics Society* 34: 711–21.

Cohen-Mansfield, Jiska. 1986. "Agitated Behaviors in The Elderly II. Preliminary Results
in The Cognitively Deteriorated." *Journal of the American Geriatrics Society* 34:
722–27.

Cohler, Bertram J. 1983. "Autonomy and Interdependence in the Family of Adulthood: A Psychological Perspective." *Gerontologist* 23 (1): 33–39.

Cole, Thomas R. 1985. "Aging and Meaning." *Generations* 10 (2): 49–52.

————. 1987. "Class, Culture, and Coercion: A Historical Perspective on Longterm Care." *Generations* 11 (4): 9–15.

Cole, Thomas R., and Sally Gadow, eds. 1986. *What Does It Mean To Grow Old? Reflections From the Humanities.* Durham, NC: Duke University Press.

Collingwood, R. G. 1959. "The Historical Imagination." In H. Meyerhoff (ed.), *The Philosophy of History in Our Time.* Garden City, NY: Doubleday.

Collopy, Bart J. 1986. *The Conceptually Problematic Status of Autonomy.* Unpublished Study Prepared for The Retirement Research Foundation.

————. 1988. "Autonomy and Long Term Care: Some Crucial Distinctions." *Gerontologist* 28 (Supplement, June): 10–17.

Colvin, D. 1989. "Fall-Safe: A Falls Intervention and Mobility Aid System for Elderly and Handicapped Rehabilitation Populations." *Technological Innovations for an Aging Population: Conference Proceedings.* Menomonie, WI: University of Wisconsin-Stout.

Coons, D. 1987. *Designing a Residential Care Unit for Persons With Dementia.* Washington, DC: Office of Technology Assessment.

Cumming, Elaine, and William E. Henry. 1961. *Growing Old: The Process of Disengagement.* New York: Basic Books.

Curtin, Sharon. 1972. *Nobody Ever Died of Old Age.* Boston: Little, Brown.

Daniels, Norman. 1985. *Just Health Care.* Cambridge: Cambridge University Press.

————. 1986. "Why Saying No to Patients in the United States Is So Hard." *New England Journal of Medicine* 314: 1380–83.

————. 1988. *Am I My Parent's Keeper.* New York and Oxford: Oxford University Press.

Dearden, R. F. 1972. "Autonomy and Education." In R. F. Dearden, P. H. Hirst, and R. S. Peters (eds.), *Education and the Development of Reason.* London: Routledge and Kegan Paul, 448–65.

Demitrack, Lucy B., and Ann W. Tourigny. 1988. *Wandering Behavior and Long-Term Care: An Action Guide.* Alexandria, VA: Foundation of American College of Health Care Administrators.

Diamond, Timothy. 1986. "Social Policy and Everyday Life in Nursing Homes: A Critical Ethnography." *Social Science and Medicine* 23: 1287–95.

Donchin, Anne. 1984. "Personal Autonomy, Lifeplans, and Chronic Illness." In L. Smith (ed.), *Respect and Care in Medical Ethics.* Lanham, MD: University Press of America, 23–44.

Douglas, Jack D. 1983. "Cooperative Paternalism versus Conflictual Paternalism." In Rolf Sartorius (ed.), *Paternalism.* Minneapolis: University of Minnesota Press, 171–200.

Dowd, J. J. 1985. "Mental Illness and the Aged Stranger." In Meredith Minkler and Carroll L. Estes (eds.), *Readings in the Political Economy of Aging.* Farmingdale, NY: Baywood, 94–116.

Dubler, Nancy Neveloff. 1990. "Autonomy and Accommodation: Mediating Individual Choice in the Home Setting." *Generations* 15 (supplement): 29–32.

Dworkin, Gerald. 1976. "Autonomy and Behavior Control." *Hastings Center Report* 6 (February): 23–28.

————. 1978. "Moral Autonomy." In H. Tristram Engelhardt, Jr. and Daniel Callahan (eds.), *Morals, Science and Sociality.* Hastings-on-Hudson, NY: Institute of Society, Ethics and the Life Sciences, 156–71.

————. 1981. "The Concept of Autonomy." In Rudolph Haller (ed.), *Science and Ethics*. Amsterdam: Rodopi, 203–13.

————. 1983. "Paternalism." In Rolf Sartorius (ed.), *Paternalism*. Minneapolis: University of Minnesota Press, 19–34.

————. 1988. *The Theory and Practice of Autonomy*. Cambridge: Cambridge University Press.

Dworkin, Ronald. 1977. *Taking Rights Seriously*. Cambridge, MA: Harvard University Press.

Engelhardt, Jr., H. Tristram. 1976. "Human Well-being and Medicine: Some Basic Value Judgments in the Biomedical Sciences." In H. Tristram Engelhardt, Jr. and Daniel Callahan (eds.), *Science, Ethics and Medicine*. Hastings-on-Hudson, NY: Institute of Society, Ethics and the Life Sciences, 120–39.

————. 1979. "Is Aging A Disease?" In Robert M. Veatch (ed.), *Life Span*. New York: Harper & Row, 184–94.

————. 1982. "Bioethics in Pluralist Societies." *Perspectives in Biology and Medicine* 26: 64–78.

————. 1986. *The Foundations of Bioethics*. New York and Oxford: Oxford University Press.

————. 1991. *Bioethics and Secular Humanism: The Search for a Common Morality*. Philadelphia, PA: Trinity Press International.

Estes, Carroll L. 1979. *The Aging Enterprise: A Critical Examination of Social Policies and Services for the Aged*. San Francisco: Jossey-Bass.

Evans, Lois K., and Neville E. Strumpf. 1989. "Tying Down the Elderly: A Review of Literature on Physical Restraint." *Journal of the American Geriatric Society* 37: 65–74.

Faden, Ruth R., and Tom L. Beauchamp. 1986. *A History of Informed Consent*. New York and Oxford: Oxford University Press.

Feinberg, Joel. 1973. *Social Philosophy*. Englewood Cliffs, NJ: Prentice Hall.

————. 1978. "The Interest in Liberty on the Scales." In Alvin I. Goldman and Jaegwon Kim (eds.), *Values and Morals: Essays in Honor of William Frankena*, Charles Stevenson, and Richard Brandt. Dordrecht, Holland: D. Reidel, 21–35.

————. 1980. "The Ideal of a Free Man." In *Rights, Justice and the Bounds of Liberty*. Princeton, NJ: Princeton University Press, 3–29.

Ferguson, C. A. 1964. "Baby Talk in Six Languages." *American Anthropologist* 66: 103–14.

————. 1977. "Baby Talk as a Simplified Register." In C. E. Snow and C. A. Ferguson (eds.), *Talking to Children: Language Input and Acquisition*. New York: Cambridge University Press, 209–35.

Ferraro, Kenneth F. 1980. "Self-Ratings of Health Among the Old and the Old-Old." *Journal of Health and Social Behavior* 21 (December): 377–83.

Fillenbaum, G. G. 1979. "Social Context and Self-Assessments of Health Among the Elderly." *Journal of Health and Social Behavior* 20 (March): 44–51.

Filner, Barbara, and T. Franklin Williams. 1979. "Health Promotion for the Elderly: Reducing Functional Dependency." In *Healthy People: The Surgeon General's Report on Health Promotion and Disease Prevention: Background Papers*. Washington, DC: U.S. Government Printing Office, 367–86.

Flathman, Richard E. 1976. *The Practice of Rights*. New York: Cambridge University Press.

————. 1980. *The Practice of Political Authority: Authority and the Authoritative*. Chicago: University of Chicago Press.

Foldes, Steven S. 1990. "Life in an Institution: A Sociological and Anthropological View." In Rosalie A. Kane and Arthur L. Caplan (eds.), *Everyday Ethics: Resolving Dilemmas in Nursing Home Life*. New York: Springer, 21–36.

Francher, J. S. 1969. "American Values and the Disenfranchisement of the Aged." *Eastern Anthropologist* 22 (1): 29–36.

Frankfurt, Harry. 1971. "Freedom of the Will and the Concept of a Person." *Journal of Philosophy* 68: 5–20.

———. 1976. "Identification and Externality." In Amelie Oksenberg Rorty (ed.), *The Identities of Persons*. Berkeley, CA: University of California Press, 239–51.

Fredman, L., and S. G. Haynes. 1985. "An Epidemiologic Profile of the Elderly." In H. T. Phillips and S. A. Gaylord (eds.), *Aging and Public Health*. New York: Springer, 1–41.

Fried, Charles. 1978. *Right and Wrong*. Cambridge, MA: Harvard University Press.

Friedman, Marilyn A. 1986. "Autonomy and the Split-Level Self." *Southern Journal of Philosophy* 24: 19–35.

———. 1987. "Care and Context in Moral Reasoning." In Eva Feder Kittay and Diana T. Meyers (eds.), *Women and Moral Theory*. Totowa, NJ: Rowan & Littlefield, 190–204.

Gadow, Sally. 1980. "Medicine, Ethics, and the Elderly." *Gerontologist* 20: 680–85.

Garfinkel, Harold. 1962. "Common-Sense Knowledge of Social Structures: The Documentary Method of Interpretation." In Jordan M. Scher (ed.), *Theories of the Mind*. New York: The Free Press, 687–712.

———. 1967. *Studies in Ethnomethodology*. Englewood Cliffs, NJ: Prentice-Hall.

Geertz, Clifford. 1973. *The Interpretation of Cultures*. New York: Basic Books.

———. 1984. "From the Native's Point of View: On the Nature of Anthropological Understanding." In R. Schweder and R. Levine (eds.), *Culture Theory: Essays in Mind, Self, and Emotion*. Cambridge: Cambridge University Press, 123–36.

Germain, Carel B. 1984. "The Elder and The Ecology of Death: Issues of Time and Space." In Margo T. Tallmer, *et al.* (eds.), *The Life-Threatened Elderly*. New York: Columbia University Press, 195–207.

Gilligan, Carol. 1982. *In A Different Voice: Psychological Theory and Women's Development*. Cambridge: Harvard University Press.

———. 1987. "Moral Orientation and Moral Development." In Eva Feder Kittay and Diana T. Meyers (eds.), *Women and Moral Theory*. Totowa, NJ: Rowan & Littlefield, 19–33.

Gilman, Sander L. 1988. *Disease and Representation: Images of Illness From Madness to AIDS*. Ithaca, NY and London: Cornell University Press.

Goffman, Erving. 1959. *The Presentation of Self in Everyday Life*. Garden City, NY: Doubleday, Anchor Books.

———. 1960. "Characteristics of Total Institutions." In Maurice R. Stein, Arthur J. Vidich, and David M. White (eds.), *Identity and Anxiety: Survival of the Person in Mass Society*. Glencoe, IL: Free Press, 449–79.

———. 1961. *Asylums: Essays on the Social Situation of Mental Patients and Other Inmates*. New York: Doubleday.

———. 1963. *Stigma*. Englewood Cliffs, NJ: Prentice-Hall.

———. 1967. *Interaction Ritual: Essays on Face-to-Face Behavior*. Garden City, NY: Anchor Books.

Graebner, W. 1980. *A History of Retirement*. New Haven, CT: Yale University Press.

Gruman, G. 1978. "Cultural Origins of Present-Day 'Age-ism': The Modernization of the Life Cycle." In Stuart F. Spicker, Kathleen M. Woodward, and David D. Van Tassel (eds.), *Aging and the Elderly: Humanistic Perspectives in Gerontology*. Atlantic Highlands, NJ: Humanities Press.

Gubrium, Jaber F. 1975. *Living and Dying at Murray Manor*. New York: St. Martin's Press.

———. ed. 1976. *Time, Roles and Self in Old Age*. New York: Human Sciences Press.

172 *Bibliography*

Gubrium, Jaber F., and David R. Buckholdt. 1977. *Toward Maturity.* San Francisco, CA: Jossey-Bass.

———. 1982. "Fictive Family: Everyday Usage, Analytic, and Human Service Considerations." *American Anthropologist* 84: 878–85.

Gutheil, Thomas G., and Paul S. Appelbaum. 1980. "The Patient Always Pays: Reflections on the Boston State Case and the Right to Rot." *Man and Medicine* 5: 3–11.

Guttman, David. 1976. "Alternatives to Disengagement Among the Old Men of the Highland Druze." In Jaber F. Gubrium (ed.), *Time, Roles and Self in Old Age.* New York: Human Sciences Press, 88–108.

Halper, Thomas. 1978. "Paternalism and the Elderly." In Stuart F. Spicker, Kathleen M. Woodward, and David D. Van Tassel (eds.), *Aging and the Elderly: Humanistic Perspectives in Gerontology.* Atlantic Highlands, NJ: Humanities Press, 321–39.

Hare, R. M. 1972. *The Language of Morals.* Oxford: Oxford University Press.

Harlow, Harry F., and Margaret K. Harlow. 1962. "Social Deprivation in Monkeys." *Scientific American* 207 (5): 137–46.

Harrell, Steven. 1979. "Growing Old in Rural Taiwan." In Pamela Amoss and Steven Harrell (eds.), *Other Ways of Growing Old: Anthropological Perspectives*, Stanford, CA: Stanford University Press, 193–210.

Hauerwas, Stanley J. 1981. *A Community of Character.* Notre Dame, IN: University of Notre Dame Press.

———. 1982. "Authority and the Profession of Medicine." In George J. Agich (ed.), *Responsibility in Health Care.* Dordrecht, Holland: D. Reidel, 83–104.

Havighurst, R. 1956. *Psychological Aspects of Aging.* Washington, DC: American Psychological Association.

Haworth, Lawrence. 1986. *Autonomy: An Essay in Philosophical Psychology and Ethics.* New Haven, CT: Yale University Press.

Hayduk, Leslie A. 1983. "Personal Space: Where We Now Stand." *Psychological Bulletin* 94 (2): 293–335.

Hegeman, Carol, and Sheldon Tobin. 1988. "Enhancing the Autonomy of Mentally Impaired Nursing Home Residents." *Gerontologist* 28 (Supplement, June): 71–75.

Heidegger, Martin. 1962. *Being and Time.* John Macquarrie and Edward Robinson (trs.), New York and Evanston: Harper & Row.

Held, Virginia. 1987. "Feminism and Moral Theory." In Eva Feder Kittay and Diana T. Meyers (eds.), *Women and Moral Theory.* Totowa, NJ: Rowan & Littlefield, 111–28.

Hendricks, C. Davis, and John Hendricks. 1976. "Concepts of Time and Temporal Construction Among the Aged, With Implications for Research." In Jaber F. Gubrium (ed.), *Time, Roles and Self in Old Age.* New York: Human Sciences Press, 13–49.

Henry, Jules. 1963. *Culture Against Man.* New York: Vintage Books.

High, Dallas M. 1988. "All In the Family: Extended Autonomy and Expectations in Surrogate–Health Care Decision-Making." *Gerontologist* 28 (Supplement, June): 46–51.

High, Dallas M., and H. B. Turner. 1987. "Surrogate Decision-Making: The Elderly's Familial Expectations." *Theoretical Medicine* 8: 303–20.

Hill, Jr., Thomas E. 1987. "The Importance of Autonomy." In Eva Feder Kittay and Diana T. Meyers (eds.), *Women and Moral Theory.* Totowa, NJ: Rowan & Littlefield, 129–38.

Hing, E. 1987. "Use of Nursing Homes by the Elderly: Preliminary Data From 1985 National Nursing Home Survey." Advance Data From Vital and Health Statistics, No. 135. Hyattsville, MD: National Center For Health Statistics, Public Health Service.

Hofland, Brian F. 1988. "Autonomy and Long Term Care: Background Issues and a Programmatic Response." *Gerontologist* 28 (Supplement June): 3–9.

———. 1990. "Introduction." *Generations* 14 (Supplement): 5–8.

Holmberg, Alan. 1969. *Nomads of the Long Bow: Siriono of Eastern Bolivia.* Garden City, NY: Doubleday.

Holmes, Lowell, and Ellen Rhoads. 1983. "Aging and Change in Samoa." In Jay Sokolovsky (ed.), *Growing Old in Different Societies: Cross-Cultural Perspectives.* Belmont, CA: Wadsworth, 119–29.

Hurka, Thomas. 1987. "Why Value Autonomy?" *Social Theory and Practice* 13 (3): 361–82.

Husserl, Edmund. 1962. *Ideas: General Introduction to Pure Phenomenology.* W. R. Boyce Gibson (tr.), New York: Collier Books.

Jameton, Andrew. 1988. "In the Borderlands of Autonomy: Responsibility in Long-Term Care Facilities." *Gerontologist* 28 (Supplement, June): 18–23.

———. 1990. "Let My Persons Go! Restraints of the Trade: Case Commentary." In Rosalie A. Kane and Arthur L. Caplan (eds.), *Everyday Ethics: Resolving Dilemmas in Nursing Home Life.* New York: Springer, 167–77.

Jeffrey, Richard. 1974. "Preference Among Preferences." *Journal of Philosophy* 71 (13): 377–91.

Johnson, Malcomb. 1976. "That Was Your Life: A Biographical Approach to Later Life." In Joep N. A. Munnichs and Winn van den Heuvel (eds.), *Dependency or Interdependency in Old Age.* The Hague: Martinus Nijhoff, 147–61.

Johnson, Mark. 1987. *The Body in The Mind: The Bodily Basis of Meaning, Imagination, and Reason.* Chicago: University of Chicago Press.

Jonas, Hans. 1966. *The Phenomenon of Life: Toward A Philosophical Biology.* New York: Dell.

Jonsen, Albert R., and Stephen Toulmin. 1988. *The Abuse of Casuistry: A History of Moral Reasoning.* Berkeley and Los Angeles: University of California Press.

Judicial Council of the American Medical Association. 1984. *Current Opinions of the Judicial Council of the American Medical Association-1984.* Chicago: American Medical Association.

Kalish, Richard. 1979. "The New Ageism and the Failure Models: A Polemic." *Gerontologist* 19: 398–402.

Kaminsky, Marc. 1984. *The Uses of Reminiscence.* New York: Haworth Press.

Kane, Robert L., and Rosalie A. Kane. 1978. "Care of the Aged: Old Problems in Need of New Solutions." *Science* 200 (4344): 913–19.

———. 1982. *Value Preferences and Long Term Care.* Lexington, MA: E. C. Heath.

———. 1990. "The Impact of Long-Term-Care Financing on Personal Autonomy." *Generations* 14 (Supplement): 86–89.

Kane, Rosalie A. 1990. "Everyday Life in Nursing Homes: 'The Way Things Are'." In Rosalie A. Kane and Arthur L. Caplan (eds.), *Everyday Ethics: Resolving Dilemmas in Nursing Home Life.* New York: Springer, 3–20.

Kane, Rosalie A., and Arthur L. Caplan, eds. 1990. *Everyday Ethics: Resolving Dilemmas in Nursing Home Life.* New York: Springer.

Kane, Rosalie A., Iris C. Freeman, *et al.* 1990. "Everyday Autonomy in Nursing Homes." *Generations* 14 (Supplement): 69–71.

Kapp, Marshall B. 1985. "Ethics vs. Fear of Malpractice." *Generations* 10 (2): 18–20.

———. 1987. *Preventing Malpractice in Long Term Care: Strategies for Risk Management.* New York: Springer.

———. 1990. "Home Care Client-Centered Systems: Consumer Choice vs. Protection." *Generations* 14 (Supplement): 33–36.

Kastenbaum, Robert. 1963. "Cognitive And Personal Futurity in Later Life." *Journal of Individual Psychology* 19: 216–22.

———. 1968. "Perspectives on the Development and Modification of Behavior in the Aged: A Developmental Perspective." *Gerontologist* 8: 280–84.

———. 1969a. "The Foreshortened Life Perspective." *Geriatrics* 24: 126–33.

———. 1969b. "What Happens To the Man Who Is Inside the Aging Body? An Inquiry Into the Developmental Psychology of Later Life." In F. C. Jeffers (ed.), *Duke University Council on Aging and Human Development. Proceedings of Seminars, 1965–1969.* Durham, NC: Duke University Press, 99–112.

———. 1975. "Time, Death and Ritual in Old Age." In J. D. Fraser and N. Lawrence (eds.), *The Study of Time I.* New York: Springer-Verlag, 20–38.

———. 1977. "Memories of Tomorrow: On The Interpenetrations of Time in Later Life." In Bernard S. Gorman and Elden E. Westman (eds.), *The Personal Experience of Time.* New York and London: Plenum Press, 193–215.

———. 1983. "Can the Clinical Milieu Be Therapeutic?" In Graham D. Rowles and Russell J. Ohta (eds.), *Aging and Milieu: Environmental Perspectives on Growing Old.* New York: Academic Press, 3–15.

Kastenbaum, Robert, Valerie Durbin, *et al.* 1972. "'The Ages of Me': Toward Personal and Interpersonal Definitions of Functional Aging." *International Journal of Aging and Human Development* 3: 197–211.

Katz, Jay. 1984. *The Silent World of Doctor and Patient.* New York: The Free Press.

Katz, Sidney, Laurence G. Branch, *et al.* 1983. *New England Journal of Medicine* 309 (20): 1218–24.

Kayser-Jones, Jeanie S. 1981. *Old, Alone and Neglected: Care of the Aged in the United States and Scotland.* Berkeley, CA: University of California Press.

Keeler, Emmett B., Robert L. Kane, and David H. Solomon. 1981. "Short- and Long-Term Residents of Nursing Homes." *Medical Care* 19: 363–69.

Kelly, M. P., and D. May. 1982. "Good and Bad Patients: A Review of the Literature and a Theoretical Critique." *Journal of Advanced Nursing* 7: 147–56.

Kemper, Peter, and Christopher Murtaugh. 1991. "Life Time Use of Nursing Home Care." *New England Journal of Medicine* 324 (9): 595–600.

Kidd, Dudley. 1904. *The Sensual Kaffir.* London: A. & C. Black.

Kiefer, Christie W. 1988. *The Mantle of Maturity: A History of Ideas About Character Development.* Albany, NY: State University of New York Press.

Kittay, Eva Feder, and Diana T. Meyers, eds. 1987. *Woman and Moral Theory.* Totowa, NJ: Rowan & Littlefield.

Kleemeier, Robert W. 1959. "Behavior and the Organization of the Bodily and the External Environment." In James E. Birren (ed.), *Handbook of Aging and the Individual.* Chicago: University of Chicago Press, 400–51.

Koch, Sigmund. 1972. "The Image of Man in Encounter Group Therapy." In J. D. Matarazzo, *et al.* (eds.), *Psychotherapy 1971.* New York and Chicago: Aldine-Atherton, 535–55.

Kohlberg, Lawrence. 1971. "Stages of Moral Development as a Basis for Moral Education." In Edmund V. Sullivan (ed.), *Moral Education.* Toronto: University of Toronto Press, 23–92.

———. 1973. "Continuities in Childhood and Adult Moral Development Revisited." In P. Baltes and W. Schaie (eds.), *Lifespan Developmental Psychology: Personality and Socialization.* New York: Academic Press, 179–204.

———. 1981. "Moral Development, Religious Thinking and the Question of a Seventh Age." In *Philosophy of Moral Development.* New York: Harper & Row, 311–72.

Komrad, Mark S. 1983. "In Defense of Medical Paternalism: Maximizing Patient Autonomy." *Journal of Medical Ethics* 9: 38–44.

Koncelik, Joseph. 1976. *Designing the Open Nursing Home*. Stroudsburg, PA: Dowden Hutchingson and Ross.

Kovar, M. G. 1977. "Health of the Elderly and the Use of Health Services." *Public Health Report* 92: 9–19.

Kupfer, Joseph H. 1990. *Autonomy and Social Interaction*. Albany: State University of New York Press.

Ladd, John. 1978. "Legalism and Medical Ethics." In John W. Davis, Barry Hoffmaster, and Sarah Shorten (eds.), *Contemporary Issues in Biomedical Ethics*. Clifton, NJ: Humana Press, 1–35.

Laird, Carobeth. 1979. *Limbo: A Memoir of Life in a Nursing Home by a Survivor*. Novato, CA: Chandler and Sharp.

Larmore, Charles E. 1987. *Patterns of Moral Complexity*. Cambridge: Cambridge University Press.

Larsen, E. B., Bernard Lo, and N. E. Williams. 1986. "Evaluation and Care of Elderly Patients With Dementia." *Journal of General Internal Medicine* 1: 116–26.

Lawton, M. P. 1981. *Environment and Aging*. Monterey, CA: Brooks-Cole.

Lawton, M. P., B. Liebowitz, and H. Charon. 1970. "Physical Structure and the Behavior of Senile Patients Following Ward Remodeling." *Aging and Human Development* 1: 231–39.

Legal Services For the Elderly. 1983. *Illegal and Questionable Terms in Nursing Home Resident Contracts: A Report to the Nursing Home Ombudsman*. Augusta, ME: Maine Committee on Aging.

Lerner, Gerda. 1986. *The Creation of Patriarchy*. New York: Oxford University Press.

Levinsky, Norman G. 1984. "The Doctor's Master." *New England Journal of Medicine* 311 (24): 1573–75.

Lidz, Charles W., and Robert M. Arnold. 1990. "Institutional Constraints on Autonomy." *Generations* 14 (Supplement): 65–68.

Lidz, Charles W., Paul S. Appelbaum, and Alan Meisel. 1988. "Two Models of Implementing the Idea of Informed Consent." *Archives of Internal Medicine* 148: 1385–89.

Lidz, Charles W., Lynn Fischer, and Robert M. Arnold. 1990. *An Ethnographic Study of the Erosion of Autonomy in Long-Term Care*. A Final Report to the Retirement Research Foundation.

Lindeman, Carol A., and Betty van Aernham. 1971. "Nursing Intervention with the Preoperative Teaching." *Nursing Research* 20 (4): 319–32.

Locke, John. 1980. *Second Treatise of Government*. C. B. Macpherson (ed.), Indianapolis, IN: Hackett.

MacCallum, G. 1967. "Negative and Positive Freedom." *Philosophical Review* 76: 312–34.

McCullough, Laurence B., and Stephen Wear. 1985. "Respect for Autonomy and Medical Paternalism Reconsidered." *Theoretical Medicine* 6: 295–308.

MacIntyre, Alasdair. 1977. "Patients As Agents." In Stuart F. Spicker and H. Tristram Engelhardt, Jr. (eds.), *Philosophical Medical Ethics: Its Nature and Significance*. Dordrecht, Holland: D. Reidel, 197–212.

———. 1981. *After Virtue: A Study in Moral Theory*. Notre Dame, IN: University of Notre Dame Press.

———. 1988. *Whose Justice? Which Rationality?* Notre Dame, IN: University of Notre Dame Press.

Macklin, Ruth. 1983a. "Problems of Informed Consent with the Cognitively Impaired." In D. W. Pfaff (ed.), *Brain and Behavior.* New York: Springer-Verlag, 23–40.

———. 1983b. "Treatment Refusals: Autonomy, Paternalism and the 'Best Interest' of the Patient." In D. W. Pfaff (ed.), *Brain and Behavior.* New York: Springer-Verlag, 41–56.

———. 1990. "Good Citizen, Bad Citizen: Case Commentary." In Rosalie A. Kane and Arthur L. Caplan (eds.), *Everyday Ethics: Resolving Dilemmas in Nursing Home Life.* New York: Springer, 60–70.

Mahowald, Mary B. 1980. "Against Paternalism: A Developmental View." *Philosophy Research Archives* 6, No. 1386.

———. 1987. "Sex-Role Stereotypes in Medicine." *Hypatia* 2 (2): 21–38.

———. "An Alternative to Paternalism." Unpublished manuscript.

Marcel, Gabriel. 1965. *Being and Having.* Katherine Farrer (tr.), New York: Harper & Row.

Mauss, Marcel. 1967. *The Gift: Forms and Functions of Exchange in Archaic Societies.* New York: Norton.

May, William F. 1975. "Code, Covenant, Contract, or Philanthropy." *Hastings Center Report* 5 (December): 29–38.

———. 1982. "Who Cares for the Elderly?" *Hastings Center Report* 12 (6): 31–37.

———. 1986. "The Virtues and Vices of the Elderly." In Thomas R. Cole and Sally A. Gadow (eds.), *What Does It Mean To Grow Old? Reflections From the Humanities.* Durham, NC: Duke University Press, 43–61.

Mendelson, Mary. 1975. *Tender Loving Greed.* New York: Vintage.

Merelman, Richard M. 1984. *Making Something of Ourselves: On Culture and Politics in the United States.* Berkeley and Los Angeles: University of California Press.

Merleau-Ponty, Maurice. 1962. *The Phenomenology of Perception.* Colin Smith (tr.), London: Routledge & Kegan Paul.

———. 1967. *The Structure of Behavior.* Alden L. Fisher (tr.), Boston, MA: Beacon Press.

Merriam, Sharan. 1980. "The Concept and Function of Reminiscence: A Review of the Research." *Gerontologist* 20 (5): 604–8.

Meyers, Diana T. 1987. "The Socialized Individual and Individual Autonomy: An Intersection between Philosophy and Psychology." In Eva Feder Kittay and Diana T. Meyers (eds.), *Women and Moral Theory.* Totowa, NJ: Rowan & Littlefield, 139–53.

Miles, Steven H. 1988. "Paternalism, Family Duties, and My Aunt Maude." *Journal of the American Medical Association* 259 (May 6): 2582–83.

Miles, Steven H., and Greg A. Sachs. 1990. "Roommates in Nursing Homes Case Commentary: Accommodating Room and Roommate Preferences." In Rosalie A. Kane and Arthur L. Caplan (eds.), *Everyday Ethics: Resolving Dilemmas in Nursing Home Life.* New York: Springer, 92–99.

Mill, John Stuart. 1978. *On Liberty.* Indianapolis, IN: Hackett.

Miller, Bruce L. 1981. "Autonomy and the Refusal of Lifesaving Treatment." *Hastings Center Report* 11 (4): 22–28.

Miller, M. 1975. "Iatrogenic and Nurisgenic Effects of Prolonged Immobilization of the Ill Aged." *Journal of the American Geriatric Society* 23 (8): 360–69.

Minkowski, Eugene. 1970. *Lived Time: Phenomenological and Psychopathological Studies.* Nancy Metzel (tr.), Evanston, IL: Northwestern University Press.

Mishra, P. K. 1983. "Proxemics: Theory and Research." *Perspectives in Psychological Researches* 6: 10–15.

Moody, Harry R. 1984a. "A Bibliography on Reminiscence and Life Review." In Marc

Kaminsky (ed.), *The Uses of Reminiscence: New Ways of Working With Older Adults.* New York: Haworth Press, 231–36.

———. 1984b. "Reminiscence and the Recovery of the Public World." In Marc Kaminsky (ed.), *The Uses of Reminiscence: New Ways of Working With Older Adults.* New York: Haworth Press, 157–66.

———. 1985. "Ethics and Aging: Old Answers, New Questions." *Generations* 10 (2): 5–9.

———. 1987. "Ethical Dilemmas in Nursing Home Placement." *Generations* 11 (4): 16–23.

———. 1988. "From Informed Consent to Negotiated Consent." *Gerontologist* 28 (Supplement, June): 64–70

Moos, Rudolf H., and Amnon Igra. 1980. "Determinants of the Social Environments of Sheltered Care Environments." *Journal of Health and Social Behavior* 21 (1): 88–98.

Moos, Rudolf H., and Sonne Lemke. 1979. *Multiphasic Environmental Assessment Procedure (MEAP): Preliminary Manual.* Social Ecology Laboratory, Palo Alto, CA: Stanford University and the Veterans Administration Medical Center.

———. 1980. "Assessing the Physical and Architectural Features of Sheltered Care Settings." *Journal of Gerontology* 35 (4): 571–83.

Morford, Thomas G. 1988. "Nursing Home Regulation: History and Expectations." *Health Care Financing Review* (Annual Supplement): 129–32.

Morgan, David L. 1982. "Failing Health and the Desire for Independence: Two Conflicting Aspects of Health Care in Old Age." *Social Problems* 30 (October): 40–50.

Mullins, Larry C., and Neil McNicholas. 1986. "Loneliness Among the Elderly: Issues and Considerations for Professionals in Aging." *Gerontology and Geriatrics Education* 7 (Fall): 55–65.

Nagel, Thomas. 1986. *The View from Nowhere.* Oxford: Oxford University Press.

Neeley, Wright. 1974. "Freedom and Desire." *Philosophical Review* 83: 32–54.

Nemore, P. 1985. "Illegal Terms in Nursing Home Admissions Contracts." *Clearinghouse Review* 18: 1165–69.

Neu, Jerome. 1975. "Thought, Theory, and Therapy." *Psychoanalysis & Contemporary Science* 4: 103–43.

———. 1977. *Emotion, Thought and Therapy.* Berkeley and Los Angeles: University of California Press.

Nisbet, Robert. 1975. *Twilight of Authority.* New York: Oxford University Press.

Norton, David L. 1976. *Personal Destinies: A Philosophy of Ethical Individualism.* Princeton, NJ: Princeton University Press.

Nozick, Robert. 1974. *Anarchy, State, and Utopia.* New York: Basic Books.

Nussbaum, Martha C. 1986. *The Fragility of Goodness: Luck and Ethics in Greek Tragedy and Philosophy.* Cambridge: Cambridge University Press.

O'Brien, Mary. 1989. *Anatomy of a Nursing Home: A New View of Residential Life.* Owings Mills, MD: National Health Publishing.

O'Neill, Onora. 1984. "Paternalism and Partial Autonomy." *Journal of Medical Ethics* 10: 173–78.

———. 1989. *Constructions of Reason: Explorations of Kant's Practical Philosophy.* Cambridge: Cambridge University Press.

O'Neill, Onora, and William Ruddick, eds. 1979. *Having Children: Philosophical and Legal Reflections on Parenthood.* New York: Oxford University Press.

Ohta, Russell J., and Brenda M. Ohta. 1988. "Special Care Units for Alzheimer's Disease Patients: A Critical Look." *Gerontologist* 28 (6): 803–8.

Pankratz, Loren, and Lial Kofoed. 1988. "The Assessment and Treatment of Geezers." *Journal of the American Medical Association* 259 (8): 1228–29.

Parsons, Talcott. 1951. *The Social System.* Glencoe, IL: The Free Press.

———. 1958. "Definitions of Health and Illness in Light of American Values and Social Structure." In E. Gartley Jaco (ed.), *Patients, Physicians, and Illness: Source Book in Behavioral Science and Medicine.* New York: The Free Press, 165–87.

———. 1975. "The Sick Role and the Role of the Physician Reconsidered." *MMFQ/Health and Society* 53 (3): 257–78.

Pegels, Carl C. 1981. *Health Care and the Elderly.* Rockville, MD: Aspen.

Pellegrino, Edmund D., and David C. Thomasma. 1981. *A Philosophical Basis of Medical Practice.* New York and Oxford: Oxford University Press.

———. 1988. *For the Patient's Good: The Restoration of Beneficence in Health Care.* New York and Oxford: Oxford University Press.

Perry, Michael J. 1988. *Morality, Politics and Law.* New York and Oxford: Oxford University Press.

Pignatello, C., M. Taylor, and P. A. Young. 1989. *The Exercise of Autonomy by Older Adults in the Home Care Setting.* Princeton, NJ: Princeton University Press.

Pincoffs, Edmund L. 1986. *Quandaries and Virtues: Against Reductionism in Ethics.* Lawrence, KS: University Press of Kansas.

Plath, David. 1983. "'Ecstasy Years'—Old Age in Japan." In Jay Sokolovsky (ed.), *Growing Old in Different Societies: Cross-Cultural Perspectives.* Belmont, CA: Wadsworth, 147–53.

Portnoi, Valery A. 1981. "The Natural History of Retirement: Mainly Good News." *Journal of the American Medical Association* 245 (17): 1752–54.

President's Commission for the Study of Ethical Problems in Medicine and Biomedical and Behavioral Research. 1983. *Securing Access to Health Care, Volume 1: Report.* Washington, DC: U.S. Government Printing Office.

Priester, Reinhard. 1990. "Leaving Homes: Residents on Their Own Recognizance." In Rosalie A. Kane and Arthur L. Caplan (eds.), *Everyday Ethics: Resolving Dilemmas in Nursing Home Life.* New York: Springer, 155–64.

Rabin, David L., and Patricia Stockton. 1987. *Long-Term Care for the Elderly: A Factbook.* New York and Oxford: Oxford University Press.

Rappaport, M., and J. B. Wood. 1989. "Financing and Home Health Agencies." *Home Health Care Services Quarterly* 10 (3/4): 131–47.

Rest, James, Douglas Cooper, Richer Coder, *et al.* 1974. "Judging the Important Issues in Moral Dilemmas of Development." *Developmental Psychology* 10 (4): 491–501.

Richards, David A. J. 1981. "Rights and Autonomy." *Ethics* 92 (1): 3–20.

Rieff, Phillip. 1966. *The Triumph of the Therapeutic: Uses of Faith After Freud.* New York: Harper & Row.

Riesman, David. 1950. *The Lonely Crowd: A Study of the Changing American Character.* New Haven, CT: Yale University Press.

Robb, Barbara. 1968. *Sans Everything: A Case and Answer.* London: Nelson.

Rogers, Carl. 1974. "Dependence and Counterdependency in Psychoanalysis and Religious Faith." *Zygon* 9: 190–99.

Rorty, Amelie Oksenberg, ed. 1976. *The Identities of Persons.* Berkeley, CA: University of California Press.

Rosenfelt, Rosalie H. 1965. "The Elderly Mystique." *Journal of Social Issues* 21 (4): 37–43.

Roth, Henry L. 1890. *The Aborigines of Tasmania.* London: Kegan, Paul, Trench, Trubner.

Roth, Julius R. 1973. "Care of the Sick: Professionalization vs. Love." *Science, Medicine and Man* 1: 173–80.

Rothman, David J. 1971. *The Discovery of the Asylum: Social Order and Disorder in the New Republic.* Boston: Little, Brown.

——. 1980. *Conscience and Convenience: The Asylum and Its Alternatives in Progressive America.* Boston: Little, Brown.

Rowles, Graham D., and Russell J. Ohta, eds. *Aging and Milieu: Environmental Perspectives on Growing Old.* New York: Academic Press.

Ruddick, Sarah. 1989. *Maternal Thinking: Toward a Politics of Peace.* Boston: Beacon Press.

Sabatino, Charles P. 1989. *Final Report: The Impact of Patient/Client Rights Regulations on the Autonomy of In-Home Care Consumers.* Washington, DC: American Bar Association, Commission on Legal Problems of The Elderly.

——. 1990a. "Client-Rights Regulations and the Autonomy of Home-Care Consumers." *Generations* 14 (Supplement): 21–24.

——. 1990b. *Final Report: Lessons for Enhancing Consumer-Directed Approaches in Home Care.* Washington, DC: American Bar Association, Commission on Legal Problems of The Elderly.

Sandel, Michael. 1982. *Liberalism and the Limits of Justice.* New York: Cambridge University Press.

Sartre, Jean Paul. 1966. *Being and Nothingness.* Hazel E. Barnes (tr.), New York: Washington Square Press.

Savishinsky, Joel S. 1991. *The Ends of Time: Life and Work in a Nursing Home.* New York: Bergin & Garvey.

Saxton, M. 1981. "Are Women More Moral Than Men? An Interview With Psychologist Carol Gilligan." *Ms.* 10 (6): 63–66.

Scarry, Elaine. 1985. *The Body in Pain: The Making and Unmaking of the World.* New York and Oxford: Oxford University Press.

Scheler, Max. 1972. *Ressentiment.* William W. Holdheim (tr.), New York: Schocken Books.

——. 1973. *The Nature of Sympathy.* Peter Heath (tr.), Hamden, CT: The Shoe String Press.

Schneider, M. D., and L. Oliver. 1987. *North Dakota Long Term Care Facilities Admission Contract Terms: Survey of North Dakota Nursing Homes.* Bismark, ND: Legal Assistance of North Dakota.

Schutz, Alfred. 1967. *The Phenomenology of the Social World.* George Walsh and Frederick Lehnert (trs.), Evanston, IL: Northwestern University Press.

——. 1970. *Reflections on the Problem of Relevance.* Richard M. Zaner (ed.), New Haven, CT: Yale University Press.

——. 1971a. *Collected Papers, I: The Problem of Social Reality.* Maurice Natanson (ed.), The Hague: Martinus Nijhoff.

——. 1971b. *Collected Papers, II: Studies in Social Theory.* Arvid Brodersen (ed.), The Hague: Martinus Nijhoff.

——. 1971c. *Collected Papers, III: Studies in Phenomenological Philosophy.* Ilse Schutz (ed.), The Hague: Martinus Nijhoff.

Schutz, Alfred, and Thomas Luckman. 1973. *The Structures of the Life-World.* Richard M. Zaner and H. Tristram Engelhardt, Jr. (trs.), Evanston, IL: Northwestern University Press.

Schweitzer, Marjorie. 1983. "The Elders: Cultural Dimensions of Aging in Two American Indian Communities." In Jay Sokolovsky (ed.), *Growing Old in Different Societies: Cross-Cultural Perspectives.* Belmont, CA: Wadsworth, 168–78.

Scott, G. E. 1990. *Moral Personhood: An Essay in the Philosophy of Moral Psychology.* Albany, NY: State University of New York Press.

Searle, John R. 1983. *Intentionality: An Essay in the Philosophy of the Mind*. Cambridge: Cambridge University Press.

Selye, Hans. 1956. *The Stress of Life*. New York: McGraw-Hill.

Sennett, R. 1980. *Authority*. New York: Alfred Knopf.

Shanas, Ethel. 1968a. " The Family and Social Class." In Ethel Shanas, Peter Townsend, *et al.*, *Old Age in Three Industrial Societies*. New York: Atherton Press, 227–57.

———. 1968b. "The Family as a Social Support System in Old Age." *Gerontologist* 19: 169–74.

———. 1979. "Social Myth as Hypothesis: The Case of the Family Life of Old People." *Gerontologist* 19 (1): 3–9.

Shanas, Ethel, and Gordon F. Streib, eds. 1965. *Social Structure and Family: Generational Relationships*. Englewood Cliffs, NJ: Prentice-Hall.

Sheehy, Gale. 1977. *Passages: Predictable Crises of Adult Life*. New York: Bantam Books.

Sher, George. 1987. "Other Voices, Other Rooms? Women's Psychology and Moral Theory." In Eva Feder Kittay and Diana T. Meyers (eds.), *Women and Moral Theory*. Totowa, NJ: Rowan & Littlefield, 178–89.

Sherman, Edmund, and Evelyn S. Newman. 1981. "The Meaning of Cherished Personal Possessions for the Elderly." In Robert Kastenbaum (ed.), *Old Age On the New Scene*. New York: Springer, 240–51.

Shield, Renée Rose. 1988. *Uneasy Endings: Daily Life in an American Nursing Home*. Ithaca and London: Cornell University Press.

Shils, Edward. 1981. *Tradition*. Chicago: University of Chicago Press.

Siegel, Jacob, and Cynthia Taeuber. 1986. "Demographic Dimensions of an Aging Population." In Allen Pifern and Lynda Bronte (eds.), *Our Aging Society: Paradox and Promise*. New York: W. W. Norton, 79–110.

Simon, Yves. 1980. *A General Theory of Authority*. Notre Dame, IN: University of Notre Dame Press.

Singer, Peter. 1979. *Practical Ethics*. Cambridge: Cambridge University Press.

———. ed. 1986. *Applied Ethics*. Oxford: Oxford University Press.

Slater, Phillip. 1970. *The Pursuit of Loneliness*. Boston: Beacon Press.

Sommer, Robert. 1969. *Personal Space*. Englewood Cliffs, NJ: Prentice-Hall.

Sommers, Christina H. 1987. "Filial Morality." In Eva Feder Kittay and Diana T. Meyers (eds.), *Women and Moral Theory*. Totowa, NJ: Rowan & Littlefield, 69–84.

Spicker, Stuart F. 1978. "Gerontogenic Meditation: Memory, Dementia and Medicine in the Penultimate Years." In Stuart F. Spicker, Kathleen M. Woodward, and David D. Van Tassel (eds.), *Aging and the Elderly: Humanistic Perspectives in Gerontology*. Atlantic Highlands, NJ: Humanities Press, 153–80.

Spicker, Stuart F., and Stanley R. Ingman, eds. 1984. *Vitalizing Long-Term Care: The Teaching Nursing Home and Other Perspectives*. New York: Springer.

Spitz, Rene. 1965. *The First Year of Life*. New York: International University Press.

Straus, Erwin W. 1963. *The Primary World of the Senses: A Vindication of Sensory Experience*. New York: Free Press of Glencoe.

———. 1966. *Phenomenological Psychology*. New York: Basic Books.

Straus, Erwin W., Maurice Natanson, and Henri Ey. 1969. *Psychiatry and Philosophy*. Maurice Natanson (ed.), New York: Springer-Verlag.

Subcommittee on Law and The Elderly. 1987. *Maryland Nursing Home Contracts: A Manual for Residents and Advocates*. Baltimore: Maryland State Bar Association.

Tagliaczzo, Daisy L., and Hans O. Mauksch. 1979. "The Patient's View of the Patient's Role." In E. Gartley Jaco (ed.), *Patients, Physicians, and Illness*, Third Edition. New York: MacMillan, 185–201.

Taylor, Charles. 1976. "Responsibility For Self." In Amelie Oksenberg Rorty (ed.), *The Identity of Persons*. Berkeley and Los Angeles: University of California Press, 281–99.

———. 1979. "What's Wrong With Negative Liberty?" In A. Ryan (ed.), *The Idea of Freedom: Essays in Honour of Isaiah Berlin*. Oxford: Oxford University Press.

Taylor, E. A. 1981. *Draft Report: Unnamed Nursing Home Investigation*. Seattle, WA: Federal Trade Commission.

Thomasma, David C. 1983. "Beyond Medical Paternalism and Patient Autonomy: A Model of Physician Conscience for the Physician-Patient Relationship." *Annals of Internal Medicine* 98: 243–48.

———. 1984. "Competency, Dependency, and the Care of the Very Old." *Journal of the American Geriatrics Society* 32: 906–14.

Tocqueville, Alexis de. 1969. *Democracy in America*. George W. Lawrence (tr.), New York: Doubleday, Anchor Books.

Toulmin, Stephen. 1981. "The Tyranny of Principles." *Hastings Center Report* 11 (6): 31–39.

———. 1982. "How Medicine Saved the Life of Ethics." *Perspectives in Biology and Medicine* 25 (4): 736–49.

———. 1990. *Cosmopolis: The Hidden Agenda of Modernity*. New York: Free Press.

Townsend, Claire. 1971. *Old Age: The Last Segregation*. New York: Grossman.

Trattner, Walter I., and W. Andrew Aschenbaum, eds. 1983. *Social Welfare in America: An Annotated Bibliography*. Westport, CT: Greenwood Press.

Tulloch, Janet C. 1975. *A Home is Not a Home (Life Within a Nursing Home)*. New York: Seabury.

Twaddle, A. C. 1979. "The Concept of Health Status." In E. Gartley Jaco (ed.), *Patients, Physicians, and Illness*, Third Edition. New York: MacMillan, 145–61.

Uhlenberg, Peter. 1987. "A Demographic Perspective on Aging." In Philip Silverman (ed.), *The Elderly as Modern Pioneers*. Bloomington, IN: Indiana University Press.

United States Bureau of the Census. 1990. *Statistical Abstract of the United States: 1990, 110th ed*. Washington, DC: Department of Commerce, Bureau of the Census.

VanDeVeer, David. 1986. *Paternalistic Intervention: The Moral Bounds of Benevolence*. Princeton, NJ: Princeton University Press.

van den Berg, J. H. 1966. *Psychology of the Sickbed*. Pittsburgh, PA: Duquesne University Press.

Van Tassel, David, and Peter N. Stearns, eds. 1986. *Old Age in a Bureaucratic Society*. Westport, CT: Greenwood Press.

Veatch, Robert M. 1981. *A Theory of Medical Ethics*. New York: Basic Books.

———. 1982. "Medical Authority and Professional Medical Authority: The Nature of Authority in Medicine for Decisions by Lay Persons and Professionals." In George J. Agich (ed.), *Responsibility in Health Care*. Dordrecht, Holland: D. Reidel, 127–37.

Vesperi, Maria. 1983. "The Reluctant Consumer: Nursing Home Residents in the Post-Bergman Era." In Jay Sokolovsky (ed.), *Growing Old in Different Societies: Cross-Cultural Perspectives*, Belmont, CA: Wadsworth, 225–37.

Vladeck, Bruce. C. 1980. *Unloving Care: The Nursing Home Tragedy*. New York: Basic Books.

Warshaw, Gregg A., James T. Moore, S. William Friedman, *et al*. 1982. "Functional Disability in the Hospitalized Elderly." *Journal of the American Medical Association* 248 (7): 847–50.

Watson, Wilbur, and Robert Maxwell. 1977. *Human Aging and Dying: A Study in Socio-cultural Gerontology*. New York: St. Martin's Press.

Weiner, Marcella Backur. 1984. "Aging as Ongoing Adaptation to Partial Loss." In Margo T. Tallmer, *et al.* (eds.), *The Life-Threatened Elderly*. New York: Columbia University Press, 31–39.

Wellman, Carl. 1985. *A Theory of Rights: Persons Under Laws, Institutions, and Morals*. New York: Rowman and Allenheld.

Wertheimer, Alan. 1987. *Coercion*. Princeton, NJ: Princeton University Press.

Whitbeck, Caroline. 1985. "Why the Attention to Paternalism in Medical Ethics?" *Journal of Health Politics, Policy and Law* 10: 181–87.

White, R. W. 1959. "Motivation Reconsidered: The Concept of Competence." *Psychological Review* 66: 297–333.

———. 1960. "Competence and the Psychosexual Stages of Development." In Marshall R. Jones (ed.), *Nebraska Symposium on Motivation*. Lincoln, NB: University of Nebraska Press, 97–141.

Whitehead, Alfred North. 1948. *Science and the Modern World*. New York: Mentor Book.

Williams, Bernard. 1973. "A Critique of Utilitarianism." In J. J. C. Smart and Bernard Williams (eds.), *Utilitarianism: For and Against*. Cambridge: Cambridge University Press, 75–155.

———. 1976. "Of Persons, Character, and Morality." In Amelie Oksenberg Rorty (ed.), *The Identity of Persons*. Berkeley and Los Angeles: University of California Press, 197–216.

———. 1985. *Ethics and the Limits of Philosophy*. Cambridge, MA: Harvard University Press.

Woodward, Kathleen. 1986. "Reminiscence and the Life Review: Prospects and Retrospects." In Thomas R. Cole and Sally A. Gadow (eds.), *What Does It Mean To Grow Old?* Durham, NC: Duke University Press, 137–61.

Yeats, William Butler. 1959. *The Collected Poems of W. B. Yeats*. New York: MacMillan Company.

Young, Patricia Ann. 1990. "Home-Care Characteristics That Shape the Exercise of Autonomy: A View From the Trenches." *Generations* 14 (Supplement): 17–20.

Young, Patricia Ann, and Martha Pelaez. 1990. "The In-Service Education Program of the Home Health Assembly of New Jersey." *Generations* 14 (Supplement): 37–38.

Young, Robert B. 1980a. "Autonomy and 'Inner Self'." *American Philosophical Quarterly* 17 (1): 35–43.

———. 1980b. "Autonomy and Socialization." *Mind* 89: 565–76.

———. 1986. *Personal Autonomy: Beyond Negative and Positive Liberty*. New York: St. Martin's Press.

Zaner, Richard M. 1981. *The Context of Self: A Phenomenological Inquiry Using Medicine as a Clue*. Athens, OH: Ohio University Press.

Zerubavel, Eviatar. 1979. *Patterns of Time in Hospital Life*. Chicago and London: University of Chicago Press.

———. 1981. *Hidden Rhythms: Schedules and Calendars in Social Life*. Chicago and London: University of Chicago Press.

Index